MW00396677

PRAISE FOR *HEALING OURSELVES*

"Dr. Shamini Jain is a visionary scientist and evolutionary leader with the energy and heart of a healer. With *Healing Ourselves*, Dr. Jain masterfully synthesizes diverse wisdom streams, weaving together scientific discoveries, ancient knowledge, and practical keys for healing to inspire and empower us to ignite infinite healing potential for ourselves, each other, and the planet. If you want to expand your consciousness and know how to best heal yourself and others, read this book."

DEEPAK CHOPRA, MD

"Shamini is that rare integration of mystic and scientist who serves as a potent bridge in a time when the divide between grounded science and ungrounded spirituality has never been more polarized. When patients have tried everything, the news isn't good, and conventional medicine has run out of options for cure, a portal of possibility opens. This is the space Dr. Jain explores in *Healing Ourselves*."

LISSA RANKIN, MD
New York Times bestselling author of *Mind Over Medicine*
and founder of the Whole Health Medicine Institute

"Dr. Shamini Jain is a pioneering voice who has dared to take us beyond common paradigms to the frontiers of a new scientific perspective—one that includes all aspects of a human being: mind, body, and spirit. *Healing Ourselves* is grounded in research, thoughtfully written, and deeply inspiring. You will read it and have hope."

EMMA SEPPÄLÄ, PHD
author of *The Happiness Track*

"Shamini Jain, a peerless scientist and spiritual adept, shines a powerful searchlight on recent discoveries concerning biofields and their profound interactions with consciousness and the natural world. This beautifully crafted book is full of scientific insights described in plain language. This is where modern medicine and healing are headed."

LARRY DOSSEY, MD
author of *One Mind*

"Between Shamini Jain's understanding of consciousness and the biofields that compose living beings, we are presented the keys to our being—and healing. Chock-full of research, this book yet leads us into the truth of the Oneness and our innate ability to realign our world, internally and externally. Yesterday's ancient wisdom becomes today's frontier of science and personal transformation, through Jain's intelligent and approachable presentation that shows how the powers of the universe—and Creation—are ours."

CYNDI DALE
author of 27 leading books on energy medicine

"Dr. Jain's authoritative review of the history, evidence, and practice of biofield science reminds us that there are answers to age-old questions about who and what we are, and that those answers—spanning both scientific and spiritual worlds—provide the keys to vibrant health and healing. I heartily recommend *Healing Ourselves* for its heartfelt wisdom and clarity."

DEAN RADIN, PHD
chief scientist at the Institute of Noetic Sciences and author of *Real Magic*

"Once in a while, there is a discovery in the biomedical sciences that opens an entirely new narrative and fundamentally reframes our understanding of the body. In *Healing Ourselves*, Dr. Shamini Jain shares such a groundbreaking paradigm. This rediscovery of the biofield within the context of Western science offers us a profound advancement: the biofield provides the long-needed linkage between the body, what we consider matter, and consciousness itself, which will lead to biomedicine ultimately surrendering its long-held firm grasp on materialism."

PAUL J. MILLS
professor of family medicine and public health, chief of the Behavioral
Medicine Division, and director of the Center of Excellence for Research
and Training in Integrative Health, University of California, San Diego

"Nature shows us how to heal. And if you want a full, nuanced, and up-to-date understanding of this simple yet profound concept, no single source will deliver it more effectively or more pleasurably than *Healing Ourselves*. Whether through clinical stories, scientific findings, lucid explanations of shifting paradigms, or personally transformative techniques, this book will inform you in all channels."

DONNA EDEN AND DAVID FEINSTEIN, PHD
coauthors of *Energy Medicine: How to Use Your Body's Energies*
for Optimum Health and Vitality and *The Energies of Love*

"The quality of your thoughts, beliefs, and consciousness produces a profound effect in your body. That's the message conveyed—in clear and convincing terms—by *Healing Ourselves*. While professionals will be intrigued by the solid science and inspiring conceptual framework, this is a straight-from-the-heart book that patients and their families will find deeply meaningful as well."

DAWSON CHURCH, PHD
award-winning author of *Bliss Brain*

"Dr. Shamini Jain is an academic, scientist, and spiritual seeker, and in *Healing Ourselves* she combines all these skills to offer a clear explanation of the human biofield and its effect on our well-being. Moving effortlessly between ancient wisdom and hard science, it's an engrossing read that explains with unusual clarity an emerging area of scientific study that is often misunderstood. I consider this a must-read for anyone who is interested in how consciousness and physicality intertwine to offer us a blueprint for health and abundance."

JILL BLAKEWAY, DACM
author of *Energy Medicine: The Science and Mystery of Healing*

"Brilliant and inspired. Evidence-based and rooted in ancestral wisdom, this is the book I have been waiting for, bridging consciousness and physiology, bringing together spirituality and health."

JOE TAFUR, MD
physician and *curandero*; author of *The Fellowship of the River*

"Dr. Jain artfully elevates our understanding of the human energy system and our potential to heal. *Healing Ourselves* goes where Western medicine is sure to someday follow and offers everyone a path to heal beyond what is offered by surgery and medication."

MIMI GUARNERI, MD, FACC
president of the Academy of Integrative Health and Medicine

"I sincerely hope everyone reads this brilliant book. Shamini Jain has emerged as a leader in the quest for a more encompassing and effective biomedicine. And she is a fabulous storyteller. The stories she has chosen to tell will help many who are looking for alternatives, especially for people who have been told by the experts that there is nothing that can be done to help them. This book can make a big difference for many people."

JAMES L. OSCHMAN, PHD
author of *Energy Medicine: The Scientific Basis*

HEALING OURSELVES

SHAMINI JAIN, PHD

HEALING OURSELVES

BIOFIELD SCIENCE

AND THE FUTURE

OF HEALTH

Foreword by Kelly A. Turner, PhD

New York Times bestselling author of *Radical Remission* and *Radical Hope*

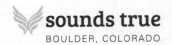
sounds true

BOULDER, COLORADO

Sounds True
Boulder, CO 80306

© 2021 Shamini Jain

Foreword © 2021 Kelly A. Turner

Sounds True is a trademark of Sounds True, Inc.
All rights reserved. No part of this book may be used or reproduced in any manner without written permission from the author and publisher.

This book is not intended as a substitute for the medical recommendations of physicians, mental health professionals, or other health-care providers. Rather, it is intended to offer information to help the reader cooperate with physicians, mental health professionals, and health-care providers in a mutual quest for optimal well-being. We advise readers to carefully review and understand the ideas presented and to seek the advice of a qualified professional before attempting to use them.

Published 2021

Book design by Linsey Dodaro
Illustrations © 2021 Meredith March

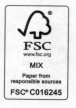

The wood used to produce this book is from Forest Stewardship Council (FSC) certified forests, recycled materials, or controlled wood.

Printed in Canada

BK05885

Library of Congress Cataloging-in-Publication Data

Names: Jain, Shamini, author.
Title: Healing ourselves : biofield science and the future of health / by
  Dr. Shamini Jain.
Description: Boulder, CO : Sounds True, 2021. | Includes bibliographical
  references and index.
Identifiers: LCCN 2020046633 (print) | LCCN 2020046634 (ebook) | ISBN
  9781683644330 (hardcover) | ISBN 9781683644347 (ebook)
Subjects: LCSH: Medicine, Psychosomatic. | Mind and body. |
  Healing--Psychological aspects. | Self-care, Health.
Classification: LCC RC49 .J35 2021 (print) | LCC RC49 (ebook) | DDC
  616.08--dc23
LC record available at https://lccn.loc.gov/2020046633
LC ebook record available at https://lccn.loc.gov/2020046634

10 9 8 7 6 5 4 3 2 1

To my Father, the finest man I know, who has always seen my highest potential and encouraged me to reach for it, while being selfless in the process. You are a true servant leader, and I can only continue to learn from your example.

This book is for you.

To my Mother, who has taught me to live life with joy and generosity—and always encourages me to uphold family and life balance no matter what the past, present, or future brings. You embody Shakti in all her divine forms.

I am grateful to be your daughter.

It has taken thousands of years, but within this century both scientists and spiritual seekers alike have once again begun to view the laws of nature and the laws of God as reflections of the same truth.

REVEREND ROSALYN L. BRUYERE

CONTENTS

FOREWORD

I first met Shamini Jain many years ago at a medical conference where we were both presenting our respective research findings. Upon seeing her speak, I instantly realized two things: (1) we were both obsessed with figuring out how so-called medical "miracles" happen, and (2) this woman knew how to pick a power suit.

While I've spent the past fifteen years studying radical remissions from the perspective of *what* these incredible survivors are doing to get well, Dr. Jain has been diligently and meticulously studying the biological and physiological mechanisms that help explain *how* these survivors get well. This book is the stunning culmination of her research to date, alongside her colleagues, who are tenured professors in major medical universities and hospitals.

Specifically, she has taken a deep dive into the world of energy and energy healing and come out the other side as a pioneer in the exciting new field of research called "biofield science." Now you may be thinking, *Hold on—you can't just make up a new field of science.* Or can you?

- Around 400 BC, scientists "discovered" that the world was round, not flat, as science had previously "proven" as fact.

- In the 1600s, thanks to the invention of the telescope, scientists confirmed that the sun was the center of our solar system, not Earth, as science had previously "proven" as fact.

- In the 1860s, thanks to the invention of the microscope, scientists "discovered" that invisible microorganisms in our air and water (not foul odors, as scientists had previously believed) caused certain illnesses.

- In the 1890s, scientists "discovered" that uranium emits radiation (even though it has always emitted it).

- In the 1900s, scientists "discovered" a new system in the body called the immune system (even though our bodies have always had one).

- And recently, in the 2000s, scientists "discovered" the biofield (even though it has always been a part of the human body and the Earth, and ancient cultures have been describing it for millennia).

So, when we look at the history of science in this way, we can see that there are really no "new" fields of science, but rather only deeper and more nuanced understandings of how our body and the world work.

This time on our planet feels similar to how it must have felt shortly before microscopes proved germ theory to be correct. During the 1840s, brave scientists like Ignaz Semmelweis and John Snow were presenting their theories about "invisible" germs, only to endure being called "unscientific" and "unsound" for suggesting such "improbable opinions." Their reputations took a hit until subsequent experiments using microscopes—conducted by Louis Pasteur and Robert Koch—vindicated their theories.

Biofield science is experiencing a similar moment in history, and you are holding in your hands one of the very first books on this new and fascinating understanding of energy and its relationship to healing. While scientists may very soon invent a new kind of "microscope" that allows them to prove the existence of the biofield indisputably, in the meantime we have the jaw-dropping studies conducted by Dr. Jain and her colleagues to ponder.

Here is just a small sampling of the new biofield discoveries you'll learn about in this book:

- We are bioelectromagnetic beings. Each of our cells has its own electromagnetic field, and these fields play a role in wound healing, tissue growth, and immune function.

- Ancient systems of medicine described the biofield as a bridge between consciousness and healing. Spiritual cultures worldwide have mapped currents of the subtle energy body, describing how these maps of energy relate to our consciousness, as well as emotional and physical health.

- Biofield-based therapies such as yoga and qigong have been shown to decrease inflammation (e.g., C-reactive protein) and help prevent diseases like cancer (e.g., by increasing telomerase activity, improving antibody responses, and more).

- Highly trained biofield healers have been shown to significantly reduce fatigue, prevent natural killer-cell decline, and normalize cortisol rhythms in cancer patients. (Amazingly, these results come from blinded studies that also offered "mock healing" to the study subjects.)

- Recently published studies at major cancer centers show that biofield healing can reduce tumor size and cancer metastases in experiments with mice—with measurable and significant effects on immune markers.

- Biofield healers have performed biofield therapies on petri dishes of both healthy cells and cancer cells. The biofield therapy improved and strengthened the healthy cells while damaging and dismantling the cancer cells—and these studies have been replicated across multiple laboratories.

It's important to keep in mind that these incredible results come simply from sending *energy*. In other words, these results are not from powerful drugs, technical surgeries, or novel immunotherapy treatments. Rather, we're talking about a simple *energy* transfer. Imagine if healing could be this powerful and also simple and side effect free. Dr. Jain's research, and that of her colleagues, indicates that this may very well be the future of medicine as we know it.

In closing, I would like to thank Dr. Jain for three things:

- First, I appreciate that she is suggesting that biofield science is **not an either/or proposition**. She is not asking us to give up our current appreciation of conventional medicine in order to embrace biofield science. We simply need to be open-minded enough to expand our current ways of thinking.

- Second, I am grateful that Dr. Jain reminds us that biofield science is **not *new*, it is ancient**. When we take the old texts of the Yogis, Jains, Hindus, and more—all of whom mapped out complex subtle energy systems—and apply those ancient texts to the novel discoveries of biofield science, it is stunning to see what humans have known all along, and what science is finally starting to measure. Biofield studies confirm what these cultures have known for millennia: the mind, body, and spirit are indeed connected, and the substance that connects them is energy.

- Finally, I am thankful to Dr. Jain for teaching us in part III of her book that we have **more power over our healing process** than the current medical model would lead us to believe. Yes, drugs and surgery are critically important, but so is living a healthy lifestyle that prevents disease in the first place. And while eating healthfully and exercising regularly are things that we all know to be important, Dr. Jain makes a compelling argument for bringing biofield exercises into our daily routines as well. The good news? The techniques she shares are free and easy to learn—and they may just change your life.

When you've finished reading this paradigm-shifting book, you can take your journey into the biofield even further at the website of Dr. Jain's nonprofit, the Consciousness and Healing Initiative (chi.is), whose mission is to bring together the best of biofield scientists and practitioners to help teach humanity how to heal through science and education.

This book marks the beginning of us collectively recognizing the biofield and, therefore, recognizing the healing power that resides within all of us. Get ready to dive into a new understanding of who we are and what is possible.

KELLY A. TURNER, PHD
New York Times bestselling author of *Radical Remission* and *Radical Hope*

INTRODUCTION

A Call for
Healing Ourselves

We are living in a time of great potential, alongside significant peril. As I write this, we're in the throes of a pandemic that has the whole world sheltering in place. First responders, particularly our health-care workers, are experiencing trauma and moral injury from witnessing coronavirus deaths and feeling responsible for choosing who of their patients get life-saving treatment and who do not, amid a largely failing health-care system. Even before the pandemic arrived, there have been serious global discussions about how best to save our planet—because we've realized that climate change is a significant reality, not a theory to be debated. Pollution and shifts in weather patterns are wreaking havoc across the world, including increasing the incidence of chronic disorders such as lung disease, which in turn affects heart health. In this changing health and environmental landscape, sociopolitical machinations seem to be pulling society into further polarizations, causing more mental and emotional distress. And with the economic fallout from the pandemic, emotional distress continues to rise within the global human family.

It's safe to say that these issues both affect and reflect the health and mental well-being of nearly everyone on the planet. Before the pandemic even occurred, the World Health Organization (WHO) and Institute for Health Metrics and Evaluation (IHME) estimated that one billion people across the world suffer from a mental, neurodevelopmental, or substance-use disorder.[1] In the United States, one in five adults—and one in six children ages six to seventeen—experience serious mental illness each year.[2] The National Center for Chronic Disease reported that mental health disorders and chronic diseases were costing the United States alone $3.15 trillion annually.[3] Because of the global nature of these problems, and because we know our emotional health affects our bodies as well as our minds and our behaviors, the United Nations has now highlighted mental health as one of its key sustainable development goals.[4]

So there is the bad news. What is the good news?

Nature shows us how to heal, once we slow down to observe and emulate it. As we shelter in place, we're noticing how profoundly nature regenerates itself. Sheltering in place has us witnessing plummeting greenhouse gas emissions and significant improvements in air quality, bringing blue skies to the most unlikely places, such as Los Angeles. Waterways such as the Ganges River (Ganga), generally fraught with industrial pollution, have begun to clear, with the water becoming potable. Animals usually rarely seen are emerging in natural places generally inhabited by humans.

During the Covid-19 *great pause,* as some have called it, we are reflecting on how we wish to evolve the systems we humans have created for a healthy, thriving life. It is time, as Native American elders say, to foster a world where humans live in right relationship with the Earth and with each other. There's never been a better time for us to envision new possibilities for a regenerative, peaceful world—and to begin to bring that world into fruition.

Today's turbulent times are causing all of us to examine what's working and not working in our systems—the ecological system, health-care system, scientific system, economic system, and even family system. Key to our next steps in improving our human systems is knowing what is possible. Given that our suffering is not only physical—it is profoundly mental, emotional, and spiritual as well—these crises point to the urgent need for us to examine, personally and scientifically, the ways we can empower ourselves to heal our human suffering instead of feeling powerless and then numbing our pain.

The good news is there is a way out. The flame that lights the path of our health and healing emanates from a source that burns brighter than the darkness of ignorance and suffering in which we have found ourselves. That's because it is a flame of unification that represents the marriage of cutting-edge scientific advancements with ancient spiritual wisdom. This marriage will finally lead us into a whole, integrated model of health and healing that we have known in our hearts, all along, to be true. Scientifically, we are finally beginning to deeply understand our ability to heal not only ourselves but also others. We have far greater power than we might have ever realized.

As we human beings evolve, so does our science. Realities doctors and scientists thought were impossible or ludicrous fifty years ago—for example, that our immune systems are connected to our brain or that our emotions influence our health—are now known to be fact, not fiction. Instead of being afraid of all microbes in our bodies as "invaders," we've learned that our immune system actually has "good bacteria" that can help us fight "bad bacteria," and that not only do our guts influence whether we get sick but that the balance of bacteria in our guts can influence our states of mind. We are discovering that our bodies and minds do not function separately but are actually parts of an interconnected whole. Discoveries in neuroscience, psychoneuroimmunology, and systems biology have helped us better understand how our thoughts, our emotions, and our sense of peace and connection deeply affect our physical health. In short, science is beginning to move away from models of disconnection and isolation into systems thinking, which fuels greater understanding in how we can heal ourselves and each other—mind, body, and spirit.

It's important to understand that when we talk about integrating science and spirituality, or expanding models of medicine, we're not throwing away conventional, allopathic medicine. This book is not an either/or proposition that suggests we need to eschew everything we've learned about medicine and health. Rather, we need to put all the pieces back together and expand further for the sake of our personal health and societal well-being. Despite what polarizing forces around us might have us think, health-care decision-making does not have to be a choice between conventional medicine and so-called alternative medicine. We need to step away from either/or thinking, which makes us feel that if we practice yoga, meditate, or practice energy healing, we might be labeled "anti-vaxxers," "anti-medicine," "anti-science," or some other ridiculous characterization. We do not have to choose spirituality over science, as if the two were really separate. We do not have to identify with camps to better foster our health. We do not need to live in fear and doubt, either. We are simply being called to honor and expand ourselves, our personal power and agency, and our full, collective understanding about health and healing. Studies suggest that human bodies and minds operate beyond the simplistic lock-and-key biochemical and receptor interactions currently thought to drive behavior. We are learning that we are not complex machines. We are bioenergetic beings completely intertwined with our environments.

Don't worry. I intend to back up these statements with science. I've been an academic for most of my life, so I am, admittedly, a data nerd. At the same time, I've always been a spiritual seeker—and have been privileged to learn from some influential healers and teachers who have opened my mind to exploring and experiencing the mysteries of consciousness and healing. It is clear to me that both aspects—empirical science and practice-based wisdom—are crucial for elevating consciousness, fostering healing, and transforming the suffering we are experiencing today individually and collectively. It's my honor to share with you what I've learned so far so that it will help you transform your own life and others' lives in positive ways.

Through my research at some of the best universities in the country and my study with some of the world's most renowned healers and spiritual teachers, I've found some key understandings about how healing works, and how we can heal ourselves, that are vital for all of us to know. I'm quite frankly shocked that most people I've met have never been told about these healing keys and have never had an opportunity to explore the practices for themselves. This book is an attempt to remedy that situation.

This book is an offering from me to you. I wrote it because I want all of us to mend our fractured understandings of healing so we can better heal our fractured selves—which are told that we are disconnected from each other, that our suffering is something "out there" that can only be fixed by a pill or some other outside treatment, and that we have no real power over our lives or our healing process. I want you to know the science behind why you have far more power to ignite your healing process and guide your life than you might have ever imagined. I also want you to be comfortable with your ability to self-heal with practical tools as you nurture and sustain yourself through your journey.

I've parsed this book into three parts. Part I, The Missing Link Between Healing and Consciousness, shares a bit of my journey to uncover the mysteries of healing and, in plain language, explores what we know about consciousness and healing from ancient spiritual traditions and modern philosophical inquiry. In the first part we also explore how groundbreaking interdisciplinary fields such as psychoneuroimmunology (my field of research) began, why they are so relevant to understanding healing, and why I think biofield science (the study of energy and information) is the bridge to help us finally, truly understand how consciousness fosters healing.

Part II, Where's the Evidence?, focuses on scientific studies of how we heal ourselves and others. We'll explore what we really know from placebo research and whether, given the data, reframing placebo from a consciousness-based perspective would make more sense. We'll go beyond the commercial hype of mind-body approaches to better understand what ancient teachings and the research data on meditation, yoga, tai chi, and similar energetic self-healing practices are really telling us about our own abilities to foster our own healing. And we'll also explore whether there's actually scientific evidence on whether we can heal others as well as ourselves, as we peer into credible, published scientific studies in biofield therapies.

Part III, The Healing Keys—with Exercises and Meditations, is a guide for you to jump-start your inner healing process. In this part, I unapologetically share both scientific data and spiritual understandings and practices. Science and spirituality are not really separate; they are simply different languages and approaches to understanding Truth. These self-healing practices draw from the scientific disciplines of psychology, neuroscience, and psychoneuroimmunology, as well as from spiritual healing wisdom.

Some of the stories I share might seem unbelievable. I'll invite you to simply suspend judgment while practicing your own clear discernment. This is the path that a true scientist, whether a PhD or a citizen scientist, walks. It's important for you, whether you're an expert or an interested person with no formal scientific background, to be able to use your own discernment to determine whether what I am sharing rings true and whether it has value for you. What I can promise you is that every study I reference is based on peer-reviewed, published scientific data. When I've referenced ancient spiritual teachings, I've done my best to choose source texts or credible translations of source-text interpretations. I've done my best not to simply cite one-off studies, but wherever possible to reference systematic reviews and meta-analyses that compile data and conclusions based not just on one study but many studies and have systematic processes that evaluate the quality of those studies as well as their outcomes. I also highlight key studies that I think tell us something meaningful and important about healing.

My wish for you is that, as you read this book, it ignites your deepest knowing—and opens the door to your connection with your full, unencumbered Self. Know that your Source is infinite bliss, that you are and will always be connected, and that you have abundant opportunities to heal any suffering you choose.

We are all on a path to healing, and we are all here to help each other as we walk the path together. It's my hope and intention that this book awakens your healing power and supports you in your journey. Namaste. Let's begin.

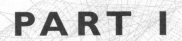

PART I

The Missing Link Between Healing and Consciousness

CHAPTER 1

The Biofield: Uncovering the Mystery of Healing

We are sorry. She only has a few months to live. There is nothing we can do."

These are devastating words no parents want to hear from a doctor about their child. When Deven and Medha's two-and-a-half-year-old daughter, Meera, their second daughter, started to show symptoms of a stomach flu that wouldn't abate, they went to the doctor immediately. They thought it might be a case of severe acidity or a chronic gastrointestinal (GI) issue. They never expected a magnetic resonance imaging (MRI) scan to reveal that their toddler had a brain tumor—and the doctors could do nothing to help her.

Deven and Medha took swift action, as any parents would. They sought the best doctors. On the doctors' recommendations, they had Meera go through radiation treatment immediately. At first, the radiation seemed to work. However, Meera developed nausea and severe ataxia (trouble walking and talking). It appeared she had swelling in her brain. A follow-up MRI showed a recurrence of a tumor in her brainstem, causing the swelling and Meera's discomfort. The tumor was malignant and positioned in such a way the doctors could not operate to remove it. There was, simply, nothing else they could do.

As you might imagine, Meera's parents were devastated. They had gone to the best cancer doctors to get answers and help, but the doctors did not know how to stop the disease and save her life.

What were their options? Accepting the doctors' words meant they were forced to watch their child painfully and slowly die in a few months. But they were not ready to accept this fate. They decided to seek other options, any safe options that would help their daughter to live and give her any chance to thrive. As they began looking for alternatives, a friend approached them.

"I'm not sure if you're open to this . . . and I know it sounds crazy," he said. "I know a healer in Tel Aviv, Israel. She was a survivor of the Holocaust." He explained that the healer, Sara, was rescued from a concentration camp as a baby after the Gestapo shot her mother. A mere twenty-four hours after the war ended and those imprisoned in the camps were liberated, an officer found Sara, still alive, under her mother's body. Sara believed this traumatic yet miraculous experience gave her healing ability. She had been healing people for many years, even from a distance. "I know it might seem like a long shot, but it might be worth a try to have Sara work with Meera," the friend suggested.

Deven and Medha considered it carefully. Although they'd never experienced distance healing before, they thought highly of their friend and knew he was trying to help them save their daughter. They were running out of options, so it didn't seem like there would be any harm in trying a session with this healer.

Sara agreed to work with Meera and explained to Deven and Medha that she would "tune in" to Meera in California from her home in Israel. She would focus on dissolving the tumor in Meera's brain every week.

Sara explained to Deven and Medha that her healing approach did not necessarily mean that she would be able to cure Meera's cancer. She shared how the process of healing was different from curing. Curing represented getting rid of a disease by specifically targeting it. Sara's healing was intended to foster Meera's inner capacity to heal herself—her body, mind, and spirit—by connecting Meera to her higher self (similar to the concepts of spirit and soul). Although Sara could not guarantee that Meera's tumor would dissolve, she had confidence that the process of healing would bring her a greater sense of peace and well-being no matter the medical outcome. Essentially,

Sara explained that curing Meera's cancer was not up to her but rather to God and to Meera's higher self.

While Sara worked on healing Meera, she asked Deven and Medha to note any changes. She also explained to them how to facilitate a balanced home environment that emulated peace, calm, and happiness to help Meera heal.

After three months of these sessions, despite the doctors' prognosis, Meera seemed better. Deven and Medha took Meera to the doctor for a brain scan. During her first follow-up appointment, the doctors said the tumor had shrunk from the size of a quarter to the size of a dime. In the next appointment, the doctors found no visible anomaly in her brainstem. The doctors were shocked. The tumor was completely gone.

"We can't understand this," they said. Meera's parents told them about the distant healer. "We've never heard of such a thing," they said. "We're not averse to believing in miracles . . . this is certainly a miracle. She's in complete remission."

Meera is still in remission today. She just celebrated her twentieth birthday with her family, well and thriving although still experiencing occasional health challenges such as seizures. She enjoys practicing classical Indian dancing and has performed in public dance troupes in California. Meera's father told me that her indomitable spirit is a lesson for all of us—she is confident, poised, and determined to live her life fully in the best ways possible.

What really happened to cause Meera's remission? Was there really a connection between those healing sessions and Meera's tumor remission, or was this just the belief of her parents? In other words, was it all just a placebo effect (a concept we'll explore in depth in part II)—and if that was the case, what does that say about the nature of healing?

Certainly Meera is not the only one to experience a "spontaneous" remission. Thousands of cases have been reported in the literature, although we still don't understand scientifically what causes these particular people to have remissions from cancer (or other ailments such as HIV, heart failure, and autoimmune diseases). We do know that in many cases, people who experience such spontaneous remissions report spiritual experiences they believe led to their healing.

Meera's case, as with all cases of "miraculous healing," leaves us with more questions than answers. The questions, which I've now devoted my work to answering through the nonprofit, the Consciousness and Healing Initiative (CHI), point to one clear challenge. Our current models of medicine fall short of understanding the depths of our human healing potential, and they are not effectively helping us solve our global health crises.

Arguably, we have never been more physically sick and psychologically miserable. The WHO reports that noncommunicable diseases such as cardiovascular disease, cancer, diabetes, and respiratory disease kill 41 million people every year (with these particular four diseases killing 80 percent of those people between the ages of thirty and sixty-nine). By 2020, the WHO estimates, chronic disease accounted for 73 percent of all deaths and 60 percent of disease burden.[1] These figures don't even take into account the increased risk of death for those with chronic diseases such as hypertension, diabetes, and cardiovascular and chronic respiratory diseases who might be exposed to viruses such as Covid-19.[2]

We also have a chronic pain epidemic, which as you might know has spurred a massive opioid addiction epidemic because our health-care system has been teaching us to numb our pain rather than heal our suffering. Although the US population constitutes only 5 percent of the global population, it consumes 80 percent of the world's opioids.[3] In the United States, costs for the current opioid crisis alone, in addition to so many lives lost, are estimated at $100 trillion since 2001. Recent reports share that these costs are continuing to rise exponentially. For example, the Society of Actuaries reports that the economic costs of nonmedical opioid use in the United States from 2013 to 2018 alone were $631 billion.[4]

Sadly, we are exporting our poor role model. The use of opioid analgesics has dramatically increased all over North America as well as in Western and Central Europe—with disastrous results.[5] In the United States, drug overdoses are the number one killer of Americans under the age of fifty.[6] No wonder we suffer from the global mental health issues we do, with more than 250 million people annually diagnosed with depression.[7]

What is causing all of this needless suffering? Why haven't we solved these health problems causing individual, societal, and global chaos of epic proportions?

The answer is fairly simple. We have been disempowered to the point where we are completely unaware of our healing potential. In fact, we doubt our abilities to foster healing in each other and ourselves, making Meera's story sound so unbelievable, especially to Western-trained medical health professionals.

Our hospital and managed-care systems are languishing from outdated, at worst, or incomplete, at best, healing practices based on disease models instead of health models. Our inability to see past disease models is keeping us from understanding and repeating the "spontaneous remissions" Meera and thousands of other people have experienced. Are these remissions indeed spontaneous, that is, without any cause? Or have we simply not understood the processes by which these seemingly miraculous healings occur? Our blind spot is definitely holding us back from creating a new model for healing this growing epidemic of disease and addiction. We need an evolution, if not a revolution, in how we best approach the way we heal.

MOVING BEYOND PATHOGENIC THINKING

Although medicine was developed to foster healing, we simply do not understand how healing works—and when extraordinary healing happens, we almost don't believe it. Why?

In order to understand why we find these miraculous stories of healing unbelievable and why we accept the current state of our global health, we have to recognize the perspectives that feed our scientific and medical systems. In our current situation, medicine is fraught with an overemphasis on physicalism and pathogenesis. Physicalism (a form of materialism) is a belief that we are essentially nothing more than our physical bodies and that all medicine must be physical in order to have effects on treating disease symptoms. Pathogenesis, in a nutshell, is the study of disease and disease progression. The Western-based pathogenic model gained credibility in the 1700s, when scientists and physicians were determined to better understand what caused disease beyond "the displeasure of the gods."[8] In the 1800s, germ theory, or the bacteriologic model of disease, helped us further understand and treat infectious disease. Because physicalism went hand-in-hand with pathogenesis at that time, the focus was on synthesizing and administering drugs (in this case, antibiotics)—such "weapons" would annihilate the "invader" germ making us sick.

They worked! Antibiotics saved—and continue to save—many people who would have died without them. Medicine evolved to be the process of getting rid of an "other" making us sick. This type of fight-the-invader thinking has not only dominated our sociopolitical structure globally for centuries but also, up until recently, our views of medicine and how the body works. We have viewed the body as a machine, with separate organs that don't necessarily talk to each other. If one of our organs has a problem, we look to physical solutions such as drugs and surgery to fix it. Although drugs and surgery certainly have their place, we're learning that other options exist as well—and that often, the body, if balanced properly, can help heal itself.

A BREAKTHROUGH IN MIND-BODY SCIENCE: THE RISE OF PSYCHONEUROIMMUNOLOGY

What happens when we expand our view of the immune system beyond that of a fighting machine to kill an "other" that lives inside of us?

Over the past twenty years, we've learned that although the immune system is designed to fight off invaders, it's far more of a cooperative, interactive, and "listening" system than we first realized. Not too long ago, we viewed the sea of microbes of different bacteria that lived within our bodies as invaders the immune system was designed to contain before they got out of control. We now know that our human guts harbor many different communities of microbes, and the optimal composition of those microbe communities can help protect against certain types of pathogens as well as help prevent cancer and heart disease.[9] Even the bacteria in our guts represent a cooperative system. We now know many of these organisms that live within us can be beneficial to our health. Our immune system not only interacts with these microbes but also with our mental and emotional states.

But consider this: Only a few decades ago, the thought that our emotions could influence our immune system was complete heresy. The field of psychoneuroimmunology didn't exist fifty years ago because we did not believe that the immune system interacted with the brain, let alone that our emotions could influence our health! Now, of course, we know that immune-brain interactions are highly relevant to understanding much of our state of disease and health—so much so that in 2017 the journals *Nature Neuroscience* and *Nature Immunology* collaborated to publish a special issue focused on the neuroimmune system. These scientific articles explore how understanding these interconnections between our immune system and brain might help us better treat disease.[10]

How did all these discoveries in psychoneuroimmunology begin? Essentially, they came from dedicated researchers who doggedly pursued their study despite ridicule and lack of support from their colleagues at the time.

Before the term *psychoneuroimmunology* (PNI for short) was even coined, there were reports of "outlandish" studies conducted by European scientists as early as the 1950s that suggested brain lesions inhibited immune reactions in guinea pigs.[11] However, these findings, and later findings that strengthened the idea of brain-immune communications, were largely ignored. At the same time, George Solomon (considered a founding father of PNI) noticed that personality and emotional factors seemed to be playing a role in rheumatoid arthritis disease expression. With his colleague Rudolf Moos, based on clinical studies and growing experimental research, he began to formally propose that the immune system and emotions were connected and that this connection had a large bearing on disease progression.[12] Further work in the late 1970s and early 1980s by European colleagues, including Hugo Besedovsky, helped to establish a growing science of immune-brain and endocrine-brain exploration.[13]

These and other early researchers of PNI, when first presenting their findings and ideas, were the laughing stock of the scientific and medical communities. Some were denied tenure. They were sometimes shut out of university laboratories for their "psychological nonsense." There was no funding to support this work, which to many seemed downright crazy. Despite the handful of promising studies and clinical observations suggesting that humans have a much deeper mind-body health connection than we realized, no one seemed to be paying any attention.

Fortunately for us, these scientists persisted—and paved a path that has had tremendous impact on our understanding of health and medicine. It was not until the definitive work of Robert (Bob) Ader and Nicholas Cohen in 1975 that people really began to pay attention.

Ader and Cohen devised a simple yet ingenious experiment—they conditioned rats' immune responses by pairing saccharin, which does not cause inflammation, with an immunosuppressant called *cyclophosphamide*, which causes gastrointestinal upset. When they gave the rats saccharin, they also injected them with the cyclophosphamide, effectively "pairing" the taste of saccharin with the drug causing the immune and intestinal distress. Not surprisingly, these rats decided they didn't like the taste of saccharin and tended to avoid it—it made them feel sick! But what Ader and Cohen found next was completely groundbreaking. They began giving the rats only saccharin and no drug. Even without the drug itself, the very taste of saccharin made the rats sick, as if they had taken the drug. In some cases, the rats even died simply from ingesting the saccharin solution. Ader even found that the responses were dose dependent—the more saccharin these rats took after being previously conditioned with the immune-altering drug, the more likely they were to have immune problems and die even when not injected with the drug. These and other subsequent studies demonstrated that rats' immune systems could be conditioned behaviorally—meaning that there had to be a link between the immune system and the brain that previously no one thought existed.[14]

With these and more studies, the field of psychoneuroimmunology began to take root. Ader and Cohen's work, building upon previous research, began to suggest that brain-immune communication, something thought impossible, is actually very much at play in our physiology and matters to our health. Further groundbreaking work in the 1980s by scientist Candace Pert demonstrated that neuropeptide receptors exist both in the walls of immune cells and in the brain. These findings paved the way for better understanding how emotions affect our immunity and opened up a related area of study in psychoneuroendocrinology.[15]

These dynamic, interdisciplinary fields of study took time to grow, but the persistent work of these early scientists paved the path for our current understanding of immune-hormone-brain interactions. Ader himself expressed the importance of systems thinking in understanding healing. It is worth exploring his original quote here:

Disciplinary boundaries and the bureaucracies they spawned are biological fictions that can restrict imagination and the transfer and application of technologies. . . . On the contrary, the evidence indicates that relationships between so-called "systems" are as important and, perhaps, more important than relationships within "systems"; that so-called "systems" are critical components of a single, integrated network of homeostatic mechanisms. To the extent that the problems chosen for study and innovative research strategies to address these problems derive from conceptual and theoretical positions, these are important issues.[16]

What was Ader saying? Essentially, he was saying that if we want to understand health, we can't understand it by boxing organs and even hormonal, immune, and central nervous systems into separate parts and thinking that understanding each part is going to drive us to understand health and healing. Rather, Ader alluded to an integrated network that fosters communication among these different "systems" and helps to guide our health. (*Homeostatic mechanisms* is simply a fancy term meaning processes that help to guide balance in a system—in this case, the mind-body system.)

What had been viewed as discrete, siloed systems of emotional states, immunity, neural functioning, and hormonal functioning now are understood as part of a larger network that regulates a person's health. Systems thinking slowly began to weave its way into Western science and medicine, helping us better understand the links between our minds, emotions, and bodies.

BIOFIELD SCIENCE: THE MISSING LINK IN UNDERSTANDING HEALTH AND HEALING

Now, even more scientists are exploring the next possible scientific breakthrough. How far might this network go? Is there truly an integrated network that guides our health, and does it relate to our consciousness? We've begun to more deeply accept and understand the influence of our emotions on our bodily function and health. Results from placebo studies also point to the power of our minds in fostering our healing. But how can we understand people such as Meera, who seemingly went into remission after working with a spiritual healer?

I and many other scientists I know are suggesting that this "network of homeostatic mechanisms" might in fact be biofields—fields of energy and information that guide our health. The network to which Ader makes reference might also be related to what indigenous cultures experienced as forces in the body, or part of the biofield.

Exploring this network of forces helps us start to uncover the crucial missing link between consciousness and healing.

Biofield science is not necessarily mysterious. The study and use of biofields includes familiar practices—such as electrocardiograms (EKGs) and electroencephalograms (EEGs). These electromagnetic readouts of the heart and brain reveal clinically important information about our state of health and are often used in medicine. But biofields extend beyond EKGs and EEGs.

Biofields can be understood as sets of interpenetrating and interacting fields of energy and information—some of them dense and electromagnetic in nature and some more subtle in nature. We are bioelectromagnetic beings. We often don't think about our bodies in terms of electricity and magnetism. We have been schooled to think of our human bodies as bags of bones, organs, muscles, liquids, and chemicals. But the truth is that humans, as with all living beings, absorb and emit energy. Our cells emit and are sensitive to electrical potentials—in fact, neural stem cells respond to electromagnetic stimulation in a way that influences how they grow and function.[17] Even our bones are piezoelectric.[18]

At present, we can explore the biofield of a cell, the biofield of a person, and the biofield of the Earth. We can also examine how biofields interact. For example, scientific studies have explored how the biofield of a person interacts with the biofield of the Earth and what that Earth-human connection can mean for our health.[19] As another example, although we are familiar with the idea that animals, such as birds, have ways to sense the geomagnetic field of the Earth to guide their migration, researchers at California Institute of Technology have now discovered that human beings have this sense as well. These researchers found, via controlled experiments, that altering the geomagnetic field actually influenced human brainwaves.[20] Not only do geomagnetic fluctuations affect our brains but also they appear to influence our heart rhythms.[21]

Although the biofield measurements we take from cells, people, and the Earth are electromagnetic in nature, all biofields might not necessarily be bioelectromagnetic. Ancient understandings of subtle energy form the basis of many medical traditions worldwide that fit under the biofield umbrella. The term *biofield* helps us bridge ancient and contemporary understandings of our bioelectromagnetic bodies and provides a common language for practice and research that explore and focus on the body's energy fields for health. The biofield perspective takes us beyond an understanding of our bodies as machines—separated from each other—to seeing them as bioenergetic beings deeply intertwined with our environments.

The biofield perspective is also informed by those who study and work with it—such that valuable contributions can be made in understanding it from many angles. For example, a researcher in bioelectromagnetics, a researcher in psychoneuroimmunology, a physicist, an energy healing practitioner, an indigenous spiritual practitioner, and a technologist all have valuable insights and perspectives on biofields that can enrich our understanding of healing.

OUR BODIES' BIOFIELDS

In addition to reading bioelectromagnetic signals from organs in our bodies as we do with EKGs and EEGs, we can also explore the biofields of cells. We've learned that cells communicate through biofields. For example, cells use their own (endogenous) electromagnetic fields (EMFs) to help guide the transport of ions and thus the electric potential in cell membranes; our bodies' EMFs also play a role in embryonic development and wound healing.[22] We can study biofields in cells, and we can also explore what happens to cell behavior when we manipulate their biofields. For example, we now know that manipulating voltage gradients across cell membranes can result in the growth of organ tissue—even neurons. Such biofield science studies are currently paving the way for new treatments in regenerative medicine in which doctors are learning how to replace diseased or damaged tissue with lab-generated tissue to help the patient heal.[23]

Biofield science also includes examining what happens if we apply biofields to our bodies, not just our cells. For example, researchers are exploring how biofield devices that use light, sound, and low-level electromagnetic stimulation on the body might help with clinical issues such as pain, wound healing, depression, and Alzheimer's disease.[24] Biofield devices' clinical effects help us to understand that we are bioelectromagnetic beings sensitive to energetic fields as well as to chemical drugs. In several cases the energetic fields themselves, even without drugs, can stimulate our healing.

In addition to bioelectromagnetic readouts of the body, nonphysical, subtle energy fields were described in ancient philosophies of medicine as key to the healing process. Although these subtle energies are less understood by scientists, they play a pivotal role in understanding biofields and healing in many ancient and modern traditions. These philosophies of subtle energy include African, Ayurvedic, Chinese, Native American, Tibetan, and other indigenous medical descriptions such as chi, ki, prana, and rlung, viewed as core components of health and healing. Naturopathic medicine calls this the *vis medicatrix naturae*. Current mind-body and spiritual approaches such as acupuncture, meditation, qigong, yoga, and others are based on understanding and shifting subtle energy dynamics to promote emotional, mental, physical, and spiritual healing. These practices using subtle energy to foster regenerative healing are thousands of years old. Healing practitioners of Healing Touch, laying on of hands, external qigong, Reiki, and many more report that they sense and work with subtle energy to foster healing. Sometimes, this *biofield healing* is called *energy healing* or *subtle energy healing*.

To better answer the question of whether subtle aspects of the biofield itself might foster healing, many biofield scientists have been examining the effects of biofield healing therapies such as Healing Touch, laying on of hands, and others—through conducting randomized, controlled clinical trials as well as research studies with cells and animals (we'll be exploring those data in detail in part II). We conduct these studies to better understand how seemingly miraculous healings, such as Meera's, happen. Stories like Meera's are more common than we realize, but we often don't hear about them because mainstream science and medicine have no explanations for them, so they are often swept under the rug as "spontaneous remissions" or "miracles" with no investigation as to why they happened.

However, instead of simply waving these miraculous stories away, we could dig deeper. We could begin to understand, through the lens of biofield science and by listening to healers, how healing happens. Then, Meera's wonderful story of healing might no longer be an anomaly but more of a commonality.

What we are discovering from biofield science so far is that biofields, whether electromagnetically measurable or not, appear to play a significant role in understanding how the body works and how it fosters and maintains health. It seems that working with biofields—whether through our own self-care practices, the use of a biofield device, or receiving biofield treatment from a trained healer—can have a tremendous role in jump-starting and amplifying our healing.

I know for some of us, this seems pretty "woo-woo." Believe me, I've witnessed the eye-rolling of many scientific colleagues when I discuss research with biofield-based healing techniques such as Healing Touch or Reiki. Some have called it nonsense or pseudoscience. But the data beg to differ—and we have the history of scientific evolution in my own research field, psychoneuroimmunology, to show how what was once thought preposterous is now common knowledge. The dedicated research by many within our nonprofit, the Consciousness and Healing Initiative, reflects this next frontier of healing research.

Scientific research into biofields is still relatively new, so its impact on science and healing is just beginning. However, as you read this book and explore the studies and stories in the subsequent chapters, as well as deepen your own felt sense of biofields through the exercises I provide in part III, I think you'll agree we are on the cusp of finally becoming awake to our human healing potential in a way we have never understood before. This new path is a true expansion of science along with understandings from ancient concepts of spirituality. It is time for us to break these unnecessary cultural silos and bridge the wisdom of our communities of Western medicine, Eastern medicine, and indigenous medicine. In chapter 2, I'll share how I discovered biofields for myself and what led me to study them.

CHAPTER 2

The Search Begins

"You want to understand healing? First heal yourself!"

The Jain nun peered at me through clear, compassionate, and no-nonsense eyes. Her retort was in response to my seemingly humble request to learn the healing secrets of our Jain tradition. Although I was slightly taken aback, I wasn't that surprised by her response. Jain monks and nuns are straight talkers—they don't pull punches, so to speak. In fact, they don't punch at all. The heart of the Jain practice is *ahimsa*, or nonviolence.

In all seriousness, many Eastern spiritual practitioners have little tolerance for teaching people who try to get fast answers without doing their own inner work first. The nun's answer reflected the hesitation many spiritual leaders feel when they are asked "deep" questions that really stem from surface understandings.

Many East Indians, right or wrong, consider us Westerners spirituality consumers. Even though I'm of Indian heritage and was raised as a Jain, I'm considered a Westerner because I was born in the United States. Some Indian sages think we're looking for quick spirituality fixes that we can purchase—or perhaps even modify to make a profit—to become gurus to the masses after completing a weekend workshop. That is likely an unfair and often untrue assessment of Westerners—as most stereotypes are—but

I'd be lying to say many in the East don't have some underlying cynicism around the commodification of spirituality. In most spiritual traditions, the ability to foster healing in another person is considered a gift or a merit that naturally arises with sincere spiritual practice, which generally takes some time to cultivate. It's not done through uncovering "secrets" and then creating products to be bought and sold.

So who was this American Born Confused "Desi" (ABCD, as we are often called), to come to India and seek the secrets of healing? Why was I asking?

My quest was sincere, but her point was well taken. I was seeking further answers, but for my personal knowledge rather than to grow wisdom. I was exploring as a scholar, not from the depths of my own personal practice. She saw through my intellectual quest and told me the truth of how I would really understand healing—to begin with myself.

Starting when I was young, I began questioning everything about reality and our role in it as human beings. I grew up in the South, and my friends were all Baptists. They were interested in my Indian heritage and the Jain practice we followed in our home, and I was interested in their traditions and beliefs. I would even go to church with them on occasion. My friends and I were eager to learn about each others' worlds and enjoyed all the innocence, play, and discoveries that come along with childhood and the exploration of different points of view.

Even though I was immersed in spirituality, I had a nagging feeling that something was missing. I was hardly an introvert but remember vividly in middle school watching all my friends running around and screaming during a birthday party, while I experienced this moment of just wanting to separate from all the happy, yet what I perceived as surface, madness. I gazed up at the vastness of the sky and the glittering stars thinking, "Is this ALL there is?"

I could not ignore the feeling that there was more to the world than what I was seeing with my eyes. Was there more to life than going to school to get good grades in order to get into a good college and make money to buy a good house and a nice car? We seemed so focused on the material world—whether it was how we looked, what others thought of us, or how much money we made. I felt there was something more to our existence than what we were told by society or what we were learning in school. At that age, however, I didn't understand what I was seeking or why I was seeking it.

This seeking feeling continued throughout my young adolescence. I was always an avid reader. I gravitated to books, not Barbie dolls (although admittedly, I was a fervent collector of all stuffed animals). When we went to the shopping mall, I would go straight to the bookstore, buy a book, and read the whole thing in an hour or two while my mom bought clothes. I also gravitated toward reading spiritual texts—particularly from the tradition I was raised in: Jainism.

If you've not heard of Jainism, you're not alone. Jainism originated and is largely based in India—and is often considered more of a philosophy than a religion. Jains do not worship a creator god. Rather, Jains believe in the existence of the human soul and believe that human consciousness has the potential to be limitless and all-knowing. Jainism bears some resemblance to Buddhism but differs in some key areas. The fundamental principle in Jainism is ahimsa, or nonviolence. Understanding that all living beings have consciousness, the potential for suffering, and a right to live, Jains vow to practice ahimsa as a means to liberate themselves and others from the cycle of birth and death.[1]

Jains follow the principle of ahimsa as devotedly as possible and are generally vegetarian or vegan, often not even eating vegetables that grow underground (because when you pull the plant from under the ground, the entire plant then dies). Often Jain monks and nuns will wear cloths on their mouths and use brooms when they walk to kill fewer organisms. Jain monks and nuns also generally only travel on foot to prevent killing organisms associated with traveling in planes, trains, and cars.

Some of the Jain and Hindu books in my parents' house had some fairly wild and unbelievable titles—*Easy Journey to Other Planets*, for example (right next to my Mom's *Cosmopolitan* magazines, equally as unfathomable to a nine-year-old). Other metaphysical books on the shelf, with less sensational titles, seemed more comprehensible.

The books explained principles from East Indian spiritual traditions, including Hinduism and Jainism, and drew from Vedic texts from the early part of the first millennium BCE. They spoke with tremendous detail about the nature of our minds, emotions, and bodies—including a "subtle world" filled with *koshas*, or subtle bodies. The books described how these bodies of energy and information flow and are unseen to most, yet they are incredibly influential on our mental, emotional, and physical states of being. The books also discussed how our physical being was completely intertwined with our consciousness and how consciousness could be considered a fundamental and unique element of each of our souls.

These concepts were totally fascinating to me (much more intriguing than the *Cosmo* articles!). So many details in these books made me wonder how the authors came up with all these insights about the human mind and body. However, when reading them, I was always left with a nagging question: How do they know this is true?

It might be helpful to provide some context here. I was a kid in the 1980s. We were all in love with *Star Wars* (some things never change, apparently), and the idea of the mind and emotions influencing the body was mostly considered the stuff of science fiction. We all loved the idea of "the Force," but we didn't really believe in it, and science certainly didn't seem to support it. Psychoneuroimmunology (PNI), the study of the connections between the mind, brain, and immune system, was still in its infancy, even within the ivory towers of academia.

As a young child, I had no knowledge of the budding field of PNI or of mind-body medicine. My father, a chemist and inventor, explained to me at an early age that "everything is understandable through chemistry and physics." Despite his strong adherence to science and the scientific method, he also had complete faith in the spiritual and metaphysical teachings of Jainism. Without any need for scientific proof, he and my mother had unshakeable belief in the existence of a soul, or eternal god-essence, that existed beyond the physical body in every living being. They believed that our thoughts, words, and deeds dictated not only our states of health but also the shapes of our lives and that subtle energy bodies reflected our states of consciousness. Despite their strong belief in the scientific method, my parents were not at all surprised that Western empirical science ignored, and often invalidated, these metaphysical and spiritual teachings.

As a family we lived many of these polarities. In the 1970s, Jain monk Sushil Kumar Muniji—one of the heads of the Jain congregation—traveled to the US to speak about Jain philosophy and ahimsa. He established Siddhachalam in Blairstown, New Jersey, as one of the places of pilgrimage for Jains in the US. The order believed that the Jains who had emigrated to the United States from India needed a place to gather and have spiritual support, so they selected Acharya ji to head this effort and gave him permission to travel by plane. Still, many Jains were actually against Acharya ji traveling to the United States. It broke tradition for him to do so (generally Jain monks and nuns travel only by foot, and on a limited basis). When Acharya ji was to board the plane for the United States, a line of Jain laypeople actually tried to block him from boarding, and he had to sneak onboard.

Acharya ji stayed with my family during his visit to the United States. During that visit, I had a formative experience that shaped my point of view but also drove home the polarities between the material and spiritual worlds I experienced as a young middle school student. My brother, then sixteen, and I, then ten, participated in a meditation session with Acharya ji, whose powerful presence and simple white dress was unlike any teachers I had encountered in the past. Acharya ji had come to the United States with a mission: he was eager to share Jain teachings and practices with the youth.

"Focus on the white light!" he proclaimed, with his eyes closed, during the session.

"What white light?" I asked, squinting my eyes shut and trying hard to concentrate. "I don't see anything."

"How do you know there is a white light?" my brother demanded. "Prove it."

Acharya ji looked at us and shook his head at what I am sure he perceived as our ignorance and insolence.

At ten, I might not have been adept at seeing white light on demand, but this experience, along with my own reflections, affirmed to me that I had a fractured education. There was no connection between an understanding of invisible worlds of inner experience (relegated to religion) and visible worlds (relegated to science).

My father and mother and most people in their generation were content to live in these two separate "scientific" versus "spiritual" worlds. I, however, could not understand why they were split. How could people make claims about reality that could not be rigorously examined by scientists? Could something as fundamental as understanding the nature of our own human consciousness really defy scientific study? I've always had an instinct to build bridges; I began to seek out models that could integrate the physical and the spiritual sides of our human experience.

In high school, as a singer, I felt the profound power of vibration during singing. I began to wonder whether there was a correspondence between what I felt when I sang and what the Vedic books described happening during chanting meditation. Could we understand our spiritual experiences by studying the principles of resonance and vibration? How did that affect our mental, emotional, and physical health? Armed with lots of questions, I left for my undergraduate studies at Columbia University, sure that I would find some answers.

I was sorely disappointed. At Columbia, I decided to study psychology and later, in my junior year, changed to the newly created major, neuroscience and behavior. I was decidedly against going pre-med (much to the chagrin of my father), but I was fascinated by the fields of psychology and cognitive neuroscience.

But it was the early 1990s, and our understanding of the brain was still limited. Even with luminaries such as Eric Kandell, who went on to win the Nobel Prize for discovering the mechanism behind our brain's neuroplasticity, at the helm of neuroscience at that time, Columbia professors emphatically explained that the brain had no plasticity (i.e., that no new neural connections were formed) after age seven. Of course, now we know this is far from the truth. But even at that time, I remember thinking, "Seriously—how can they say the brain is static by seven years of age?" How could these brilliant neuroscientists studying the dynamics of biology and the brain for decades be so sure of that black-and-white conclusion, when there were such limited data?

At that time, neuroscience focused on examining local brain regions associated with function. Most scientists seemed content to report on which part of the brain lit up during a particular cognitive task, and that was the end of the scientific discussion. There appeared to be no interest in exploring the mind because researchers assumed that anything we called *mind* was simply the result of brain activity (a view still strongly held by many scientists today). There also seemed to be no interest in connecting the brain to the rest of the body—in fact, my honors research thesis advisor, a brilliant cognitive neuroscientist, once remarked, "I don't understand why people are still studying things like heart rate and skin conductance. I mean, we have the brain!!" Cognitive neuroscience had all these new, fancy imaging tools, and the idea of studying the body beyond the brain fell out of favor. And questions surrounding the mind-body connection, or consciousness, were just too messy.

YEARNING FOR MEANING

I left Columbia with my bachelor's degree, excited to leave New York City and explore new horizons at Stanford University, where I was fortunate to be offered a position as a research assistant in studies that examined brainwave function in people with schizophrenia and Alzheimer's disease at the Palo Alto veterans' hospital. I had a strong yearning to do research that would make a difference in people's lives and was excited to be involved in a project in which scientific breakthroughs could help patients.

However, my naive idealism was soon humbled by the realities of academia. The focus seemed more on strategizing how to get the next grant and less focused on research that would directly benefit patients. I remember the day I was placing electrodes on a person with Alzheimer's for a routine study, and he asked me plainly and sincerely, "Is this research going to help me?" I realized that it wasn't going to help him directly, and at that moment, I knew it was time for me to move on to an area of study that would more directly help patients.

I wanted to find an academic "home" that would, at the very least, tolerate and possibly encourage my deeper questions surrounding consciousness and health. However, it was difficult to find academic programs and professors who shared the same interests—so I did my best to educate myself in the interim while enjoying life in the Bay Area. I took courses at the University of California–Santa Cruz in organic chemistry and the physics of music. I started to work with an incredible voice teacher. He encouraged me to expand my abilities as a coloratura soprano and really explore how guiding the voice through my body could result in the creation of different tonalities and expansion of vocal range. At the same time I was exploring the reaches of classical Western singing, I began exploring sound healing on my own. I was personally feeling the power of running resonant vibrations through my body during singing and wondered how music and sound could be better used for healing. Surely, sound healing and mantras were connected to vibration, which influences our consciousness and our state of health. The scientist in me wanted to understand how we might actually measure the relationship between consciousness, vibration, and health, but I could not think of a model experiment or situation to study.

Until I had my first Reiki session—which literally changed my life.

AN UNEXPECTED BREAKTHROUGH

Juno (not her given name) was your typical twenty-something Santa Cruz vagabond healer. She had dreadlocks and a stray dog with "abandonment issues" who went everywhere with her. She was dabbling in several healing arts while figuring out her next move. She was friends with one of my roommates and introduced me to this "energy therapy" called *Reiki* she had learned. She said it was relaxing but different from meditation. I was curious to know what it was all about and asked her for a session.

When Juno arrived to give me the Reiki session, the ritual of it all struck me right away. She came dressed in flowing white clothes, lit incense, and said prayers. She put on a CD of soothing instrumental music. She invited her "guides" in and invited me to say any prayers or invite any guides I had to come into the process. The rest of the session would be held in silence, so I could simply be with the energy. I have to admit at that point I had no idea what to expect, and I didn't expect much. But I trusted nothing terrible would come of it, so I said a prayer and hopped on the table fully clothed to see what would happen. I figured, at the very least, I'd have a nice nap.

Juno began placing her hands lightly on different places around my body, starting with my head. I felt some warmth and tingles at first and then noticed a constricted sensation when she got to my belly area. All of a sudden I felt all this tight energy moving around in my stomach, and it was surprisingly painful (generally people don't feel pain during a healing session).

I realized that this moving around of stuck energy seemed related to certain thoughts and memories. I would literally have thoughts flash by as the tight sensations loosened in my body, and the thoughts seemed related to fears and anxieties that I realized I needed to let go of. My mind traveled to previous and current situations in which I was giving my power away by not being truthful with myself or others about how I was feeling. It was a pretty heavy session, but what I got out of it was profound. It seemed as if whatever was coming through Juno's hands was bringing up not only tightly held sensations in my belly but also tightly held emotions and thoughts in my mind—memories and issues that I had not wanted to deal with but that I realized in those moments continued to make me feel sad and powerless. I now felt empowered to look those issues in the eye and to get past them in a way I hadn't felt before. I experienced all of this without even talking about it to Juno during the session.

How was this possible? We weren't talking at all, and yet these emotions and thoughts seemed to come up only when she put her hands on certain areas of my body, particularly my belly. That was interesting to me because I had been suffering from acid reflux since I was a child (I had not told her this). Now, I was feeling this energy moving from my belly all around my body when Juno was touching me. Was this movement related to the descriptions of prana and the "vital energy body," the "life force superhighway," I had read about in our Vedic texts as a child? The light went on in my mind.

I realized that the profound experience I had during this introductory Reiki session had opened the door to being able to study the relationship of consciousness and health. As a singer, I had witnessed the power of using sound and vibration internally to shift my own state of consciousness but was struggling to understand how, for example, I could research the power of music and sound to heal another person without simply resorting to describing changes in brain areas that occurred with music perceptions.

Although it seemed obvious that sound and music affected people's bodies and brains, vibrational healing seemed more profound than simply having brain areas light up. Certainly, the Vedic texts described the effects of sound on subtle bodies and spiritual states of consciousness—but it was unclear how to study this scientifically. I was particularly interested in measuring the effects of the sound vibrations and exploring how these vibrations could affect another person's state of consciousness and health, from the spiritual to the physical levels. But how could I guarantee that a person could feel or hear a sound vibration emanating from the music player or singer? How could I determine how the vibrations themselves might foster healing?

With the Reiki session, I realized that *here* was a vibration, although subtle, that I could literally *feel* in my body. Moreover, the subtle vibrations I was feeling in my body were connected with something Juno was doing, along with what I was thinking, remembering, and feeling. The energy flowing through her to me was literally bringing to light all of these issues that needed to be healed on the emotional, mental, and perhaps even physical levels. But what was the nature of this energy? Where was it coming from? And could it really affect healing, down to the cellular level?

Perhaps it was what scientists called a *placebo*? I couldn't rule out that possibility. The session had a lot of elements we know facilitate a placebo response—ritual, relationship, and expectation. For example, a clear ritual was set before I even got on the table (candles, incense, white clothing, soothing music). I had a friendly relationship with Juno and trusted her, and we know positive relationships with health providers can affect our nervous system. Expectation plays a huge role in outcomes as well—although I didn't know what to expect, I was eager to learn more about Reiki and was certainly hoping something interesting would happen. All of these factors could have created responses in my mind and body. (I've investigated placebos in depth—see chapter 5 for my take on them.)

But how could I explain the relationship between the thoughts and emotions I was having and the sensations I was feeling when she had her hands on my belly? The session was conducted in silence. I did not tell her what I was feeling when she was working on me, and she hadn't given me any indication that belly pain or even feeling subtle sensations in my body would happen. What was actually going on during the healing?

Reiki healers say that they are actually conduits for Reiki, which they define as "universal life energy" (some say "divine life energy"). They, like many healers, prepare for the healing session by "grounding and centering" (a practice we will explore later in this book). Then, they literally do their best to get their minds out of the way and allow this universal/divine energy to flow through their hands into the person being healed. From a Reiki healer's point of view, then, Juno was not doing the healing; she was acting as the conduit for healing to take place.

What was this universal life energy, and how did Reiki healers access it? Could anyone do it? Or was the belief of the healer influencing the belief of the patients and engaging them in some sort of hypnotic process that altered their perception? Did Reiki and similar therapies actually influence health and healing?

I left that Reiki session realizing I had lots of inner emotional clearing to do—and at the same time, my mind was even more curious and determined than ever to find scientific answers to what I had just experienced. If this was truly a way for people to heal others, it ought to be scientifically investigated; and if useful, it should be brought to more people to help them heal as well. I searched for university professors researching healing from the perspectives of neuroscience and psychoneuroimmunology, but I couldn't find any. I couldn't find any recent research on biological changes from healing approaches such as Reiki. It seemed as if most of the research in healing was conducted by nurses decades ago, and they were not mentoring students in PhD research programs.

But this work seemed so profound and important—a field ripe for discovery and understanding about human health. Certainly there were some luminary thinkers synthesizing data and perspectives on energy healing—such as James Oschman, Daniel Benor, and Richard Gerber, who shared data in areas including bioelectromagnetics and studies with plants, humans, animals, and cells. But these researchers were not at universities actively conducting clinical studies of healing in patients, where my heart really lay. I decided that when I went to graduate school, I would start to study healers and the effects of energy healing on health outcomes. Now, I just had to find a mentor at a good university who would understand and support me to pursue this research.

As it turned out, I was fortunate to find and learn from several fabulous mentors who supported my passion and direction. My first foray into healing research began with Gary Schwartz and Iris Bell at the University of Arizona, in collaboration with that university's Center for Integrative Medicine. A father of behavioral medicine, Schwartz had made many breakthrough discoveries himself at Harvard and Yale Universities in psychophysiology and had a history of mentoring successful academics. (For example, he mentored Richie Davidson, a well-known meditation and neuroscience researcher at the University of Wisconsin–Madison, as well as Shauna Shapiro, a well-known author and mindfulness researcher at Santa Clara University.)

Schwartz, an innovative scientist, had a jovial, nurturing demeanor and provided a safe environment in which his students could explore questions about consciousness and human nature from an open, scientific viewpoint.

Whatever students chose to focus on for their project, he supported them wholeheartedly. He fostered their education as scientists and was always interested to hear their ideas. He always made time to spend with his students and treated each of them with kindness and respect. But what made him special as a mentor was not simply his innovative thinking—he supported his students to do the research they most wanted to do.

Mentoring students to let them study what they wish is actually somewhat rare in academia. I had learned that in most labs, students were treated a bit like factory workers; mentors often assumed students would adopt their research interests and work on specific projects for which mentors had received funding and needed help. This helped keep the academic machine chugging away. Professors wrote the grants in research areas they had staked out as their own in order to get tenure and received relatively inexpensive labor in exchange for mentoring graduate students who helped to conduct their studies. Graduate students, in turn, got a small stipend for their work (much better than paying for graduate school out of their own pockets) in exchange for the training and published journal articles they needed to advance their careers. They just didn't always have the freedom to pursue their own ideas. This academic model is efficient but not necessarily one that fosters innovation, particularly in young scientists.

Schwartz's lab, on the contrary, was a haven for innovative thinking.

Not long after I joined his lab, as synchronicity would have it, Schwartz received funding to conduct a study on Reiki healing. Knowing my interests, he invited me to join the research team. I was thrilled to be the junior scientist on the project and looked forward to doing actual research on this healing therapy. Little did I know I was about to have another profound experience with Reiki—one that would help me to further understand the links between what I had learned from Vedic texts on the connections between consciousness, biofields, and healing.

CHAPTER 3

Consciousness: Modern and Ancient Perspectives

Armed with a blossoming understanding of this energy therapy called Reiki, I was excited about studying its effects. I began to read up on this particular form of healing and learned that Reiki is an ancient Japanese form of spiritual healing founded by Mikao Usui, a Buddhist monk and doctor in Japan in the early 1900s. Usui had a spiritual awakening that guided him to create this healing practice. He began treating people in Japan with Reiki. Eventually, another Reiki practitioner named Hawayo Takata brought Reiki to the United States. Many forms of Reiki are practiced worldwide, but the "mother," or traditional, form of Reiki is Usui Reiki, sometimes also called Usui Shiki Ryoho (see reikialliance.com/en for more information). Traditional Usui Reiki was the form we planned to study.

We had several meetings with Reiki healers and the research team as we discussed possible study designs. Our research team was eager to conduct a placebo-controlled trial that would compare trained Reiki healers with "sham" Reiki healers. The sham healers would be giving a placebo therapy. The real Reiki healers were not so keen on this design, explaining to us that "energy is everywhere" and that the sham healers would be moving energy as well, although they would not be trained, and thus the study would not be controlling for energy per se. They felt that in order to better study and understand Reiki, it would be useful for us to experience it more fully. They requested that all of us on the research team be initiated into Reiki Level 1 with the head teacher.

I was curious about this request. What was this "initiation," and why did they feel we needed it? Wasn't I already initiated, having received a Reiki session in the past with Juno? After all, I had experienced a movement of energy in my body when she worked on me.

Our Reiki healers explained that receiving a Reiki session was not the same as receiving a Reiki initiation. Part of the Reiki training process involves a deliberate transmission of energy through the healer to the student using a specific Reiki ritual. At a certain point in the training, the teacher, a Reiki master with decades of practice and teaching, would place her hands at the top of each student's head (opening their crown chakra) and, using specific symbols and prayer, "attune" or "initiate" the students to the Reiki energy so that it always stayed with the initiate after the training sessions were over.

Well, that sounded pretty far out. Attuning my crown chakra with energy that stayed with me for the rest of my life? Was it really possible? My parents wondered: Was this dangerous or some sort of voodoo or cult thing? My scientific mind figured it was harmless. Obviously, these healers followed a ritualistic belief system, and it was important to them that we did this so that we could understand what they did in their healing and therefore study it better. And who was I to judge the validity of what they were saying? Wasn't that what the research was for, after all?

To my surprise, the Usui Reiki initiation ended up being quite profound for me. I remember it quite clearly more than twenty years later. After explaining the history and basic concepts of the Reiki practice on the first day of the two-day training, the teacher prepared us for this initiation. She asked us to visualize in our mind's eye our "highest power," a god or symbol that represented the Divine to us.

When I closed my eyes, I saw the image of Mahavira Swami, the last enlightened soul in Jainism to teach the Jain way (similar to the Buddha). As I held the image of Mahavira in my mind, the Reiki teacher placed her hands above my head. I immediately experienced an enormous bliss I had never felt before in my life, one that lasted for some time. The feeling was as palpable as the joy one feels when holding one's child for the first time, or of being completely in love with someone. In this case, I felt in love with the entire world. I remember sitting on the outside sidewalk during our lunch break, simply wrapped in this blissful feeling of unity for what must have been an hour, grinning from ear to ear, registering a bit of surprise from the teacher as she noted my experience and waited for me to "come down." None of us had expected my reaction.

Needless to say, after that experience, I was even more eager to study this process of Reiki healing and understand what it was. The Reiki initiation, like my first Reiki session, was palpable for me. In both cases, I could feel the energy running through my body, and it was associated with strong emotions. In the case of the Reiki initiation, I wondered whether somehow the process hadn't initiated some sort of neurotransmitter release associated with my state of bliss. Certainly, neurotransmitters such as serotonin and oxytocin are associated with love and blissful emotions. But how could that spiritual process, involving no drug, no needles as in acupuncture, not even any physical movement, and no specific expectations initiate such a strong feeling of bliss?

I realized I didn't understand Reiki and these energy therapies deeply, and in order to better study them, it would be useful to explore the practice a bit further. I took Reiki Level 2 and began working with relatives on occasion, curious as to whether I could use Reiki to reduce pain or feelings of discomfort. But I was really acting as an investigator of healing. I was curious about the outcome but did not want to assume anything about the effects of the practice. After all, I had chosen the path of an objective scientist and felt I couldn't be biased by totally buying into the Reiki path if I was going to study it.

If you've had a Reiki session or initiation like I've had or heard similar stories, you might wonder: Do these therapies really have any basis in the history of medicine and healing—or are they simply "new age" therapies? Reiki and other *biofield therapies*, as we scientists often call them, beg lots of questions, none of them easily answerable. Although many people might consider these biofield or energy healing approaches fairly new, the truth is they have been used for millennia in many different cultures. Other examples of currently practiced biofield therapies include Healing Touch,

Johrei, laying on of hands, Therapeutic Touch, Pranic Healing, external qigong, and many more.

But truthfully, the historical basis of biofields extends beyond even these therapies. Concepts relating to biofields such as chi, prana, qi, and others are used in current mind-body practices such as qigong, tai chi, yoga, and many forms of meditation. Entire medical systems such as Ayurveda, Chinese medicine, Tibetan medicine, and others are based on ancient understandings that what we modern scientists call the *biofield* is a key interface between consciousness and healing.[1]

WHAT'S CONSCIOUSNESS GOT TO DO WITH IT?

Oh no—I've invoked the dreaded "C" word! Consciousness? What the heck is that anyway, and how does it relate to biofields? This is where many of my scientific colleagues throw up their hands in exasperation. "Shamini! We barely understand what a biofield is," my friend and colleague Richard Hammerschlag, a longtime acupuncture researcher, said. "Do we really need to now invoke and discuss concepts of consciousness to understand a biofield? That means we are dealing with two unknowns! Not good for research!"

It might not be easy or convenient, but I have stood my ground on this point with Hammerschlag and other colleagues now for years, and the more he reads about consciousness from luminary philosophers such as systems scientist and two-time Nobel Peace Prize nominee Ervin Laszlo, the more he begrudgingly agrees with my assertion that we must bring consciousness into the discussion to understand biofields and their effects on healing.[2]

So what do we mean by consciousness? Let me start by acknowledging that entire books, volumes of books, weeklong annual conferences, and even university courses are devoted to this subject, and therefore what I am sharing with you here is not at all comprehensive but reflects both current and ancient understandings of consciousness.

Consciousness can mean different things to different people. Many have implied that consciousness means "awareness" of our environment. This suggests, of course, that we could be only partially aware of certain things and therefore experience them in an unconscious way. Consider influential psychologists such as Sigmund Freud and others who popularized terms such as *conscious*, *unconscious*, and *subconscious* in their descriptions of the mind, emotions, and psychotherapy. These psychologists described how our experiences shape our emotions and emotional reactions. They also described how often our emotions could be "subconscious"—that is, we might not be fully aware of them, but they drive our behavior—sometimes in ways we don't recognize. This suggests that what we call *awareness* is related to consciousness and how we behave.

Carl Jung expanded the view of consciousness as it related to the human psyche and psychotherapy. He described the personal conscious and unconscious as well as a "collective unconscious." He based his theory on the idea that we inherit archetypical patterns of personality that represent our unconscious drives and influence our behavior.[3]

Others take a slightly different view of consciousness, explaining it as our subjective experience of our environment. For example, consciousness explains my experience of seeing, smelling, and tasting a red apple. This felt, conscious experience is often called *qualia* in Western philosophical explanations. Qualia is, quite simply, our subjective experience.

The term *qualia*, made popular by American philosopher C. I. Lewis in the late 1920s as a description of properties of sensory data, has now been expanded so that in modern-day philosophy of consciousness, it refers to our perceptions, mood states, and body sensations.[4] My experience of energy running through my body during the Reiki session and initiation would be considered a type of qualia—regardless of whether it can be measured. Others experiencing a Reiki session might not feel the same thing; they might have a totally different experience and, therefore, different qualia.

What explains why I have the type of felt experience I have and why someone else might have a different felt experience? To give a more mundane example, even the experience of drinking a cup of coffee might not be exactly the same for you and for me. Although certain brain networks responsible for smell, taste, temperature sensing, and even memories would likely become active for both of us, our actual experience of drinking the coffee might not be exactly the same. The experience of qualia is a fundamental aspect of our consciousness. It is simply our phenomenological experience of the world around us, and there is no "right" or "wrong" or need for validation of what it is. It is the experience itself.

In 1995, Western philosopher David Chalmers helped catapult modern philosophical perspectives of consciousness forward with a provocative thesis. He deliberated on how the experience of qualia relates to the "hard problem" of consciousness.[5] The hard problem is that of how our subjective experiences, such as consciousness, connect with physical changes, such as brain and body processes. The hard problem is basically a reframing of the mind-body problem, which has plagued philosophy, science, and medicine for centuries. The basic "problem" is this: How does my experience, which is subtle and seemingly nonphysical in nature, relate to physical matter, such as my body? For example, how can shifts in my conscious state of being affect my healing?

An example of the hard problem, or the mind-body problem, was my experience during the Reiki initiation. When the initiation took place, I strongly felt the experience in my body—the moving of energy from my head into my body—and these feelings were closely associated with a state of spiritual and emotional bliss. Yet there was no physical cause—I wasn't touched, I didn't take a drug, I wasn't meditating before the initiation began, and I wasn't doing a physical yoga asana. Yet through the initiation I was immediately brought to a profound and healing state of consciousness. Others have felt similar effects during biofield therapy sessions. What explains that experience?

Chalmers asserts that we can consider the functional relationships of conscious experience with body processes an "easy" problem. For example, we can explain processes such as attention, information integration, and communication by measuring brain and body processes. We can conduct computational modeling and look at brain mechanisms and neural networks to understand how we pay attention, learn, and communicate ideas.

However, according to Chalmers and others, a person's actual state of experience, or qualia, is difficult, if not impossible, to explain via body processes and brain mechanisms. The hard problem asks: What explains the state of experience I have when drinking a cup of coffee, watching a sunset, or feeling pain? Why should any of these stimuli give rise to the types of qualia they do?

Many neuroscientists assert that the experience of consciousness simply emerges from complex brain activity. For example, many philosophers and scientists who have materialist views of consciousness believe it arises from matter—more specifically, they argue that all conscious experience arises from the cellular activity in our brains.[6] Chalmers and others argue this explanation is not sufficient, and not all matters of consciousness can be explained by brain processes. They would relate the brain and body to a radio or TV set, meaning that our brains and bodies filter and broadcast consciousness that exists outside the TV. The TV does not have the program actually inside of it; it has to connect to a signal to show the program. The internet is not located inside your computer; you connect to a Wi-Fi signal to access it. Similarly, a nonmaterialist view of consciousness is that subjective conscious experience, or qualia, does not depend on the brain and in fact does not arise from the organ of the brain. The brain is a receiver, not the ultimate creator, of consciousness.

Chalmers and others suggest the term *consciousness* should be reserved for our actual subjective experience, or qualia. They suggest using the term *awareness* instead to describe the "easy" problems such as attention, discrimination, information integration, and communication, which can be explained by computational and neural network solutions. Chalmers might claim that although we could trace the neural pathways that correspond to awareness functions such as attention and communication, there is no physical brain correlate for the actual experience of consciousness itself. He suggests consciousness might be a fundamental and irreducible part of nature that exists outside of our brains and bodies, as with the law of gravity.[7] "Now I have to say I'm a complete atheist; I have no religious views myself and no spiritual views, except very watered-down humanistic spiritual views, and consciousness is just a fact of life; it's a natural fact of life," he wrote.

As you can imagine, Chalmers's thesis set off a lively debate and discussion among philosophers worldwide about the nature of consciousness and how it could be studied. Chalmers's thesis provided a springboard for scientists and philosophers to finally come out to other colleagues about discussing and exploring the science of consciousness.

This movement toward the scientific study of consciousness was quite significant considering that not long before, consciousness was thought to defy scientific exploration and was, quite frankly, denied discussion in academic settings. Through Chalmers's and others' work, academic centers for the scientific study of consciousness such as the Center for Consciousness Studies at the University of Arizona, the Center for Consciousness Science at the University of Michigan, and the Center for the Explanation of Consciousness at Stanford University are now thriving. Societies such as the Society for Consciousness Studies and international conferences such as the Science of Consciousness conference, held annually, are fostering dialogue among differing schools of thought on consciousness who approach the hard problem in different ways. The camps on consciousness are mind-boggling in themselves: reductionism, eliminativism, panpsychism, epiphenomenalism, mysterianism, and many more "isms!"

Some philosophers say there is no hard problem because there is no such thing as consciousness—that what we are calling *consciousness* is just a term to make sense of how our brains and bodies view the world. Others claim that consciousness exists but can only be broken down into brain mechanisms. Still others claim that the problem of consciousness can never be solved by current scientific methods or by the human mind because our minds are too limited to grasp the complexities of consciousness outside of our minds.

Why should we care about how we understand and experience consciousness? At some level, I will admit, I am a pragmatist. Although I grew up in academia, I've also grown tired of pedantic papers that assert one view of anything (including consciousness) over another for the sake of simply winning a logical argument. However, I do believe these discussions on consciousness are helpful and important to understanding the healing process, including why biofield therapies such as Reiki work. I believe we need to study more deeply how consciousness, however people view it, affects healing. Understanding that consciousness is intimately related to our health and well-being and uncovering how consciousness fosters healing are vital for the evolution of medicine.

CONSCIOUSNESS: ANCIENT PERSPECTIVES

Interestingly, some of the theories of consciousness rekindled by Western philosophers have been reflected in ancient medical and philosophical teachings for millennia.[8] These teachings, thousands of years old, not only explored the nature of consciousness but also provided frameworks for helping us better understand how consciousness could play a role in healing.

For example, East Indian philosophical systems, including Advaita Vedanta, Kashmir Shaivism, and others have put forth theories of consciousness and reality that stem from first-person experiences of spiritual practitioners. Through the processes of logical inference and empirical exploration, these experiences were developed into frameworks to guide practice—similar to other indigenous traditions.[9] This evolution contrasts with that of most Western philosophies, which generally discard first-person experiences as having no bearing on theory development. Instead, they rely solely on mental formulations and logical arguments that to some degree they consider devoid of actual first-person experience. (Consider, for example, the Descartian phrase "I think, therefore I am." An experience-integrated framework might sound more like "I am, therefore I think.")

East Indian theories of consciousness share similarities with Chalmers's view of consciousness: They also posit that consciousness is irreducible—that is, it cannot be broken down into small parts and does not arise from brain processes or from any physical matter or cause. However, these ancient philosophies of consciousness go a bit further in their descriptions. These and other ancient philosophies describe aspects of consciousness associated with human perception, cognition, and awareness that we can call aspects of "little c" consciousness. In addition, they also describe a primordial, universal, "big C" Consciousness that is by its nature not bound to any physical form and yet gives rise to all experiences and all forms. Essentially, these philosophies claim that this "big C" Consciousness gives rise to matter, not the other way around. This "big C" Consciousness is a formless Oneness.

Vedantic philosophy is not the only wisdom tradition that has described formless Oneness. Similar concepts have been described in many spiritual traditions, including the "void" or emptiness in Buddhism and the "Tohu Bohu" as described in the Old Testament, suggesting that several spiritual traditions refer to a similar, if not the same, base of "big C" Consciousness.[10]

From the Advaita Vedanta perspective, Consciousness is eternal and nonphysical, and it gives rise to everything. This philosophy is based in nonduality—the view that everything, even matter, comes from a nonphysical Consciousness and that, ultimately, all "little c" consciousness is part of a unified, unchanging Consciousness. The unchanging, eternal Consciousness, called *purusha*, is the ultimate reality, but the world of illusion in which we find ourselves (*maya*) makes all that is conscious in the physical world appear as separate, embodied forms of consciousness (*prakriti*).

Advaita Vedanta and other spiritual traditions explain that as we deepen our spiritual practice, we begin to penetrate maya, this veil of illusory appearance, and we begin to realize that our "little c" consciousness is actually a reflection of "big C" Consciousness. Through spiritual practice, we begin to realize that we, the many "little c" conscious beings, are in fact all deeply connected to each other and the "big C" Consciousness.

Many would equate this "big C" Consciousness with Divinity or God, and indeed Vedic tradition describes it as such. It is called *Brahman*, and its qualities are described as *sat-chit-ananda*—a formless, naturally eternal, all-knowing, blissful, absolute Consciousness.[11] At times during meditative or other spiritual practice, one may experience states of *samadhi*, transient experiences of the qualities of this absolute Consciousness in which one makes contact with Oneness. There are different levels of samadhi, some of which are characterized by ecstatic bliss.[12]

I believe I had a taste of a samadhi state during my Reiki initiation.

What keeps us from being in this divine, blissful Consciousness at all times? From the Vedic point of view, it is natural not to be in this divine, blissful Consciousness all the time because we are human. As human beings, at our core, we are truly reflections of this Divine Consciousness, but we get in our own way of experiencing it. This is because we live in a cycle of feeling both attachment—being drawn to things we want—and aversion, avoiding unpleasant or painful experiences we don't want. Both attachment and aversion set up causal chains (which some call *karma*) that lead us to experience the pinnacles of both worldly joy and immense, debilitating suffering. Because we are constantly living in a push-pull world, driven by our roller coasters of emotions, mental machinations, desires, and repulsions, we are simply not aware of the eternal, divine Consciousness that lives within us and in everything. We are not in a place of pure awareness to witness this

Divine Consciousness. Humans are therefore reflections of nonduality or Oneness, living in a dual world of illusory separation, or maya.

From a Vedic spiritual point of view, the path of healing is realignment with our Divine Consciousness. Through the healing process, we come to know the depth and breadth of who we truly are as conscious beings, and, as a result, we experience shifts in our emotional, mental, and physical well-being. From this vantage point, healing is not simply curing a disease or mitigating a pesky symptom—although that is possible and certainly does happen. Healing is about reconnecting with the deepest core of who we are—beyond our fears, worries, excitement, to-do lists, medical problems, and roles we play in the world. Healing is that path that realigns us with what many would call our soul, or spirit, or God as well as with the nature that surrounds us. From this view, the path of healing aligns with the path of spiritual liberation as well as social and ecological harmony.

All of this might sound abstract to some people. How do we entertain the idea of, or better yet experience, an all-knowing Consciousness, and how does that augment our healing process, exactly? If consciousness is nonphysical, and yet we experience healing on spiritual, emotional, mental, and physical levels, how does that work? What is the intermediary between consciousness and healing?

We can get a clue from the practices suggested by ancient philosophical and spiritual teachings around the globe. They literally prescribed as well as described spirit-mind-body practices including centering prayer, meditation, and yoga to help one to more fully develop and realize the deeper aspects of Consciousness within one's self—called *being one with God, spiritual liberation,* or *self-realization.*[13]

Because these ancient spiritual philosophies were also holistic, they described how spiritual progression affected mental, emotional, and physical functioning and health. Key to understanding the interconnection between the spirit, mind, and body is the existence of subtle bodies, including a vital energy body, described as being a conduit for life force and a key player in how consciousness affects healing.[14] Subtle bodies and vital energy are part of what we now call *biofields* in Western science.

As we dive deeper in chapter 4 into ancient East Asian perspectives on subtle energy bodies, we will see how these spiritual traditions described how to work with subtle energy for spiritual development and healing. As we progress through this book, we'll also uncover how current scientific research in subtle energy healing (also called *biofield healing*) is paving the way for a true revolution in understanding health.

CHAPTER 4

Subtle Bodies and the "Stain of Vitalism"

I reflected deeply on the transformative experience I had during my Reiki initiation. It was similar to the Reiki session with Juno, in which I could feel the energy in my body. But during the initiation with the Reiki master, my consciousness temporarily moved to a whole new level—to a feeling of bliss and deep connection with the world. My state of consciousness literally shifted when the Reiki master placed her hands above my head—but I didn't understand why or what she had done. She explained that she had used specific symbols to direct energy down through the top of my head, or crown chakra, into my body. This is a protocol all Usui Reiki masters do when initiating a person into the universal life energy. Through her intentional use of symbols, she seemed to open a floodgate of energy that shifted my consciousness.

How could such a thing happen? In order to understand what she was saying, I had to understand the link between consciousness and this subtle energy. I couldn't find any scientific research articles explaining what I had just experienced, although the literature contained accounts about similar bliss states reached through meditation. But I was not practicing meditation when this happened. It seemed to be directly related to something the Reiki master had done. I realized I'd have to figure out my experience by listening to the healers and exploring what ancient cultures had said about this energy and how it relates to consciousness.

As we explored in chapter 3, ancient cultures described an eternal, blissful, and all-knowing Consciousness. Deep down, this is reflected in our essential nature as humans. Beyond our cultural conditioning, life experiences, likes, and dislikes, we are all part of a unitary Consciousness. In the so-called illusory world of maya, however, we appear to be separate parts and pieces of this Consciousness. The *leela*, or divine play, at hand is to dance back to our true nature, to return to the divinity that exists within us through spiritual practice. When we connect more deeply with the nature of Consciousness, we experience profound shifts in our states of being. We move closer to mental, physical, emotional, and social harmony. This is the process of healing. During my Reiki initiation, the Reiki master's intentional use of sacred healing energy and symbols opened my energetic channels to experience a greater connection with that energy. I believe my feelings of bliss in that moment were because I felt a greater connection to Divine Consciousness.

Even if we fully accept these ancient spiritual teachings, want to embark on this healing path, and perhaps wish to help others to heal, many questions arise. Exactly how can connecting with Consciousness foster healing on these emotional, mental, and physical levels? What is the bridge that connects Spirit with these changes on the physical plane? How can one person's consciousness possibly heal another person?

Ancient cultures and even more recent cultures had their own way of explaining the energetic bridge between consciousness and healing. Although Western scientists now use the term *biofields* to explain fields of energy and information that guide our health—including *bioelectromagnetic* fields and more *subtle* fields—terms and concepts related to what we call the biofield have been used for thousands of years across cultures worldwide. They described the "missing link" between consciousness and healing as a type of vital life force.

Ancient and more modern cultures have shared deep philosophies and practices involving the knowledge of vital life force and its relationship with healing. Chinese, Japanese, Egyptian, Maori, Hebrew, Lakota, and Yoruba cultures used terms such as chi, ki, ka, mana, ruah, ni, and ase, respectively. Later in Western civilization and philosophy, vital life forces were described as elan vital, orgon, bioplasmic energy, and more.[1] The understanding of vital life energy plays a role in modern holistic medicine practices today; for example, one of the core principles in naturopathy is *vis medicatrix naturae*, which refers to the body's intimate connection with nature and innate ability to heal itself.[2]

Although the descriptions of these forces and their interaction with the mind and body vary in their descriptions and depth, they all reflect a philosophy of vitalism—the belief in an animating force that distinguishes living beings from nonliving matter and helps foster the health of our bodies and minds.

What is the nature of this "life force"? How does it affect our minds and bodies, and how would it serve as a bridge between consciousness and healing? How does this life force affect the physical body, and how does it interact with consciousness?

ANCIENT TEACHINGS: SHAKTI, THE MIND, AND SUBTLE BODIES

Although the precise origin of the vital life force concept is difficult to determine, this force and its relationship to consciousness have been described by numerous spiritual traditions. Many traditions described the relationship of consciousness with subtle energy as well as subtle energy bodies beyond the physical body that served to transmit vital life force and reflect informational patterns related to our consciousness.

How does subtle energy relate to mind, consciousness, and spiritual liberation? In many spiritual traditions, systematic processes are described to guide the spiritual aspirant to recognize and work with subtle energy to expand consciousness and gain spiritual wisdom, if not spiritual liberation. In the Tantric traditions, for example, Consciousness in its absolute form is described as *Shiva*, a formless Oneness that is pure, unmanifested Being. Complementarily, *Shakti* is the energy behind Consciousness, the power behind all creative action, and the force that fosters manifestation of all worldly forms. Shiva is considered the cosmic masculine principle and Shakti the cosmic feminine. Tantric tradition describes the complementary and codependent nature of Shiva and Shakti in the world we live in. Put simply, Shiva without Shakti has no power to manifest, and Shakti without Shiva is directionless. One must cultivate and unite both aspects (being in choiceless awareness, and allowing for full flow of the creative force) for spiritual growth and liberation.[3]

Buddhist teachings have likened these principles to the mind and the vital force by noting that vital energy is like a blind horse, whereas the mind is like a lame rider. One must unite the mind and the vital force to achieve spiritual growth—and by doing so, we unite the cosmic masculine and feminine aspects of consciousness that lie within each of us.

How do we realize the Shiva and Shakti within us? Ancient texts describe how certain mind-body practices (which I detail in chapter 6) can allow one to better understand the nature and power of this vital energy in our bodies, which is related to the cosmic creative force of Shakti. Through these practices, one learns how to use the mind to recognize and guide the energy through one's body to foster healing, gain spiritual insight, and even provide a pathway to enlightenment through completely relinquishing the conditioned mind.

How does one feel and guide this vital energy through the body? Tantric, Vedic, and other texts describe *koshas*, or subtle energy bodies; *chakras*, or subtle energy hubs; and *nadis*, or subtle energy pathways by which this creative vital force can travel in the body to bring harmony and health as well as deeper spiritual growth. The descriptions of subtle bodies in ancient traditions help us to understand how our ordinary consciousness—all the way down to our thoughts, words, and deeds—influences our mental, emotional, and physical states of being. They also help explain extraordinary states of consciousness, including human beings' abilities to foster healing in each other through the use of vital life force. The vital energy body is where bodily life force energy (prana) moves and has its effects on physical and mental well-being.

Deep descriptions of subtle energy bodies as bridges between the gross physical body and subtle workings of consciousness were described as early as the fourth and fifth centuries BCE, for example, in the Taittiriya Upanishad.[4] This is not the only literary source that describes such subtle energy bodies; these bodies have been described in numerous cultures. In this chapter, we'll explore the East Indian descriptions, knowing that they are only one culture's description of these bodies as they relate to healing.

Ancient Upanishadic texts from the sixth century BCE describe humans as having five types of koshas (sheaths).[5] These koshas are described as being nested so that they permeate and interact with each other. The bodies are also described as being increasingly subtler in substance, although all of them are considered material. The most "gross," or most material in nature, is *annamayakosha*, the physical sheath. Following the physical body is the *pranamayakosha*, or vital energy sheath, slightly more subtle than the gross physical body. Next, in a higher grade of subtlety, is the *manomayakosha*, the mental sheath or body of thought; then the *vijnamayakosha*, the wisdom body or body of awareness, discrimination, and intuition; and finally, the *anandamayakosha*, the causal sheath or body of bliss.[6] The texts state that for most humans, the four more subtle sheaths are not generally perceivable, but adept spiritual practitioners can have awareness of these bodies and actually use them in their spiritual development process or healing of others. Similar subtle bodies are described in ancient Jain as well as Tantric texts, although their descriptions and names are slightly different.[7]

Jain teachings as well as several forms of yoga and tantra have similar concepts of the subtle bodies. For example, they describe the subtle body as being composed of the *tejas sarir* or *taijas sarir*, translated as the fiery body; and the karmic body, called the *karma sarir*. Jains describe the fiery body as forever entwined with the karmic body in humans, and together they are called the *suksma sarir*, or subtle body.[8]

KARMA AND ITS ROLE IN HEALING

Jains describe dynamic karmic patterns that occur through our thoughts, words, and deeds as existing in the subtlest of all the bodies—karma sarir, or the karmic body. Karma refers to the law of cause and effect. The understanding is that everything we do, say, and think creates an information pattern in the karmic body that gives rise to an action tendency. For example, repetitive acts of violence toward the self or toward others create a specific pattern in the karmic body. So do repetitive acts of kindness. Each action drives us toward another specific action, whether we execute that action by thought, word, or deed. Karma is thus created through chains of action. Everything we do mentally, emotionally, and physically creates a particular response—stored as an informational pattern—and influences our consciousness.

Jains believe the soul's force is filtered through karmic patterns and radiates through the suksma sarir, or subtle body, in vibrations. In Jainism, these subtle vibrations are called *adhyvasyaya*, and they are described in both physical and mental terms, meaning that these karmic emanations affect both our bodies and minds.[9]

Ultimately, the karmic emanations created by our thoughts, words, and deeds filter through our vital energy body and shape how our moment-to-moment consciousness affects our mental, emotional, and even physical state. This dynamic interaction between the soul's consciousness; the vital body; and day-to-day mental, emotional, and physical experience has been depicted in figure 4.1 by a Jain scholar.

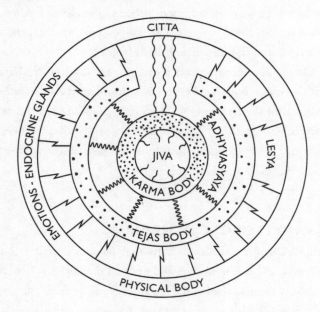

Figure 4.1. Simplistic model of Jain descriptions of *jiva*, the embodied soul; *citta*, consciousness; and their expression through the karma body, tejas body, and physical body (the subtle bodies). From the Jain perspective, the rays of consciousness from the soul interact with the karma body and give rise to *adhyvasyaya*, or subtle vibrations. These karmic emanations influence the makeup and dynamics of the tejas (fiery) body and affect physical and emotional functioning. These vibrations also reflect a person's psychospiritual state and can be "read" by a person's *lesya*, or spiritual coloring (similar to what some healers call the *aura*). Narayan Lal Kachhara, "Philosophy of Mind: A Jain Perspective," *US-China Education Review* (2011).

Through this framework, we come to understand how we experience our consciousness—which by its fundamental nature is all-knowing, eternal, and blissful—as limited. Because of our human tendencies to engage in attachment, avoidance, and ignorance, we create karma through our thoughts, words, and deeds. Continued habit patterns create karmic patterns in the subtle body. These karmic impressions are called *samskaras* in Sanskrit and give way to *vasanas*, or habit patterns, essentially formed by our conditioning or continuous chain of samskaras. In this way, karma is seen as nothing more than habits—which we can change. When we are aware of our habit patterns and can change them—all the way to recognizing, disrupting, and releasing the karmic pattern—we have liberated ourselves fully from a habit that does not serve us. This literally frees up energy in our system—which helps us heal and move toward greater well-being—ultimately by experiencing the well of our being, Divinity itself.

Putting together these teachings on consciousness and the subtle body, I realized that the feeling I had during the Reiki initiation was a taste of the well of my being. From the Vedic and Reiki points of view, during my Reiki initiation the Reiki master opened a major hub of energetic connection through my crown chakra. The Reiki master facilitated movement of life force energy through an intention to open my consciousness and allow energy to move more freely through me, connecting me and aligning me with a deeper sense of soul connection. There was some movement, some "unblocking"—some would say a reshifting of karmic information—that happened in order to allow me to have a stronger sense of God-consciousness.

THE SUBTLE BODY: A BIDIRECTIONAL COMMUNICATION SYSTEM

It's important to understand that in these ancient traditions, the subtle body is not described as just an amplifier of karmic patterns. It can be considered a bi-directional communication system between the physical body and the soul—a gateway that connects Spirit with our physical, emotional, and mental being.

Pranamayakosha, or the vital energy body, is described as the closest to the gross physical body in terms of its makeup. It has been described in most depth in terms of its relationship to the physical body and health. Several Upanishadic texts, estimated to be written in the early part of the first millennium BCE, describe in detail the "energy anatomy" within the pranamayakosha that serves to connect the mind with the body.[10] They describe major energy hubs, called *chakras*, related to elements and qualities of consciousness as well as more than 70,000 vital energy channels through which prana flows in the body, called *nadis*. Knowledge and use of the chakras, nadis, and their corresponding *marma* points are incorporated into whole-systems medical approaches such as Ayurvedic medicine. In Ayurvedic medicine, prescribed practices such as *asanas*, specific yoga postures; *pranayama*, breathing exercises; meditation; massage; and others are given to facilitate the flow of energy through these subtle energy channels to guide health.

Ayurvedic and yogic texts describe the flow (or lack of flow) of energy through chakra, nadi, and marma points as relating to health states we often ascribe to our nervous and endocrine systems. Similar descriptions of energetic pathways and relationships to organ systems exist in other indigenous, whole-health systems of medicine. An example is the explanation and use of acupuncture points and meridians in Chinese medicine. At this point we cannot say that the nadi system and the meridian system are describing the same pathways, although comparisons have been made, and some healers posit that these concepts are more similar than different.[11]

Several spiritual teachers and scholars suggest that shifts in subtle energies as felt in chakras influence the release of hormones, noting that the location of chakras correspond with the location of main endocrine glands. These teachers and scholars also posit that movement and flow of subtle energy in nadis relates to lymph and nervous system activities. It's important to note that these might be more modern interpretations of ancient texts.[12] Also, keep in mind that the descriptions of subtle channels corresponding with the physical nervous system does not mean that these subtle channels are parts of the physical nervous system. In other words, we haven't found a plethora of hard research evidence that would reduce our understandings of the nadis to the lymph system directly or evidence that chakras are just labels for endocrine glands. Little empirical research to date truly explores the relationship of the subtle pathways and physical anatomy, although some scholars describe anatomical correlates of what they believe to be subtle energy channels. For example, some research groups in China have proposed that novel circulatory structures called Bonghan ducts correspond to acupuncture meridians.[13] Although there is still much to discover, the descriptions of these subtle energy hubs and channels are notably similar to our descriptions of the nervous system.

How might these nadis, or subtle energy channels, connect with nervous system functions? Yogic texts describe two main nadis (one called *ida*, which refers to the "moon" and "passive" energies, and the other called *pingala*, which refers to the "sun" and "active" energies) that have qualities corresponding to the parasympathetic ("rest and digest") nervous system and the sympathetic ("fight, flight, or freeze") nervous system, respectively. The ida nadi, described as being on the left side of the body, reflects the feminine energies of receptivity and stillness. These aspects of consciousness correspond with the known functions of the parasympathetic nervous system to foster relaxation of peripheral muscles and slow the heartbeat, providing the body the stillness it needs for restoration. The pingala nadi, said to be on the right side of the body, is described as mobilizing or activating masculine energy—corresponding with the sympathetic nervous system, which among other actions increases our muscle activity and heartbeat, readying our bodies to think and act swiftly as needed. The *sushumna* nadi is described as the "central channel," from which kundalini energy, or the "sleeping serpent," arises to foster greater spiritual development and ultimately liberation of the soul from its bondage to the physical body. This central channel appears to correspond with the spinal column. These are only three of the main nadis described; many more are discussed in detail in both the source texts and their more modern translations and interpretations.

These texts also describe the importance of pranayama, working with the breath, to direct subtle energy through the nadis in order to reduce mental, emotional, and physical toxicity and bring one toward a greater state of harmony. Interestingly, and not surprisingly, yogic pranayama exercises meant to balance the ida and pingala energies have been found to stimulate the vagus nerve (the main "driver" of the parasympathetic nervous system) and foster the body's natural healing response.[14] Modern-day teachers such as Wim Hof draw from pranayama exercises as well as other ancient

Tibetan Buddhist exercises, such as Tummo, in their teachings, now gaining popularity in the West. The practices are altered slightly from their original indigenous sources, and the explanations for these alterations (and related fields, including mindfulness) are that stripping the religious and spiritual meanings away from the practices are ways to make them more accessible (and thus more marketable) to all.

If we approach the wisdom within these spiritual traditions with openness, as opposed to feeling we need to strip away teachings from their original cultures and appropriate them to the dominant culture, I believe we'll understand the depths and subtleties of the original teachings for ourselves. As an example, we'll learn that prana is not just one type of energy. Yogic and Ayurvedic texts delve deeper into the aspects of prana as it relates to bodily functions and describe the different aspects of *vayus*, or prana in the body, that need to be balanced for mental and physical health. Related Buddhist teachings and later Tibetan medical texts also described how *rlung* (in Tibetan), or imbalances in these aspects of subtle energy, could lead to mental and physical disorders. The practice of balancing these subtle energies for mental and physical health is very much alive in these traditions of medicine today.[15]

Clearly these teachings and practices have influenced modern-day teachers of mind-body wellness. Did these ancient descriptions of subtle energy also influence Western theories of science and medicine? We can surmise that even the founders of psychoneuroimmunology (PNI) recognized that these ancient descriptions of mind-body connection were linked to their pioneering efforts. For example, PNI leader George Solomon, who witnessed the impact of emotions on disease progression in his patients, wrote in one of his papers: "It appears that we have come full circle in recently recognizing that the mind is integrally related to the body and that it is impossible to separate one from the other. Interestingly, this is the very premise of many Eastern religions and systems of medicine. For example, in Ayurvedic medicine, an ancient proverb holds that 'the forces in the body are in harmonious relationship with the environment' (Charaka Samhita, English translation, 1949)."[16]

"THE STAIN OF VITALISM":
WORLDVIEW CLASHES IN MEDICINE

It's important to recognize that this ancient model of consciousness and its relationship with subtle energy and health is just that—a model that attempts to integrate the experience of adept practitioners and scholarship through empirical and logical inquiry to help make sense of the world around us. It does not necessarily mean that the model is "right" and all other models are "wrong." Modern medical models are created through empiricism and clinical experience and are ultimately derived from the dominant cultural worldview, which attempts to explain who we are and what the nature of the world around us is.

Ancient models of medicine are similar in that they derive from both scholarship and spiritual experience—however, the worldview that underlies both the scholarship and experience is different from the current view in Western medicine today. Western medicine as it is mostly practiced today relies on a worldview of separateness and physicalism—that disease comes from a pathogen that is "not me" and that I can only use physical medicine to get rid of it.

In Ayurvedic, classical Chinese, and Tibetan medicine, for example, the models of healing are based on worldviews that regard consciousness as a fundamental and unitary aspect of the universe. Spiritual experiences are not considered separate from physical experiences, but rather both nonphysical spirit and physical matter derive from the same original substance—Consciousness. The body has an innate ability to heal itself, and this process can be encouraged by fostering proper flow of life force energy, which serves as a conduit between consciousness and physicality.

These Eastern teachings provide an underlying model to help us better understand and explore communications between the spirit, the body, and our environment. Disease is considered disharmony that might exist within one's self or between one's self and his or her surrounding environment. Thus, healing is not about curing yourself from something that is "not you" but understanding the patterns that might be causing you disharmony and therefore illness. The vital life force is a bridge that allows the healer—ultimately you—to better understand the nature of that disharmony and bring harmony back to your system.

Vitalistic thinking was not just inherent in Eastern medical systems. It influenced Western medicine for centuries. For example, Greek philosopher Aristotle's (384–322 BC) theories of matter and form (called *hylozoism* or *hylomorphism*) described his views of the soul (which he considered "form") as the life-giving force of the physical body (which he considered "matter").[17] Aristotle saw the soul and body, or form and matter, not necessarily as separate but as essential aspects of living beings.[18] Aristotle's philosophies greatly influenced Western medicine and science, including the work of Greek physician Galen and others.

Many iterations of vitalistic theories in basic science followed between the sixteenth and twentieth centuries in Western biology and medicine. For example, when eighteenth-century physician Caspar Fridrich Wolff (considered the father of epigenesis) observed the emergence of structures out of the hearts of developing chick embryos, he enthusiastically proposed "a principle of generation, or essential force [*vis essentialis*] by whose agency all things are effected."[19] Evolving definitions of vitalism continued to pepper Western science and medicine in the seventeenth, eighteenth, nineteenth, and twentieth centuries through other doctors, biologists, and chemists, including Johann Friedrich Blumenbach, Louis Pasteur, Hans Driech, and others.

However, the Western scientific and medical community never met vitalism with blind fervor. Many scientists from the seventeenth century onward, influenced by the mind-body dualism of Réne Descartes as well as Isaac Newton's physics and mechanistic theory, viewed vitalistic theories as mere "hand-waving" or "lazy science" to account for effects that likely had a mechanistic explanation simply not yet uncovered. For example, in the early 1800s a premise of vitalistic theory in terms of its relation to chemistry was that organic material could not be synthesized from inorganic material. The idea was that only living things could create organic material. However, an experiment conducted by Friedrich Wohler, who used inorganic compounds to create an organic compound—urea—refuted this claim based in vitalism (and also founded organic chemistry).[20] Although skeptics credit this experiment as having completely disproved vitalism, other scientists and historians note that this experiment's discrediting of vitalism as a whole is simply a myth.[21]

The debate over the existence of the vital force continues to be contentious in Western science and medicine. In our current zeitgeist of materialism, which dominates the very fabric of society today, *vitalism* is simply considered a dirty word, and those who even suggest the presence of vitalism in science or medicine are, at best, seen as ignorant and inept and, at worst, seen as knowingly misleading others through pseudoscience and called "quacks." Francis Crick, the famed codiscoverer of DNA structure, for example, is also known for his famous quote: "And so to those of you who may be vitalists I would make this prophecy: what everyone believed yesterday, and you believe today, only cranks will believe tomorrow."[22]

Cranks, indeed? It certainly appears today that a scientist calling another scientist a "vitalist" is the ultimate smear campaign.[23] Yet the fundamental understandings that surround these ancient spirit-mind-body practices examined for their health benefits today—such as acupuncture, biofield healing, craniosacral therapy, meditation, qigong, tai-chi, yoga, and more—are rooted in vitalist thinking. Underlying their practice are philosophical theories of unitary consciousness, subtle energy bodies, and experiences of vital life force. As we'll explore in detail in part II, more and more scientific research suggests that these mind-body and subtle energy therapies are beneficial for a number of ailments, including for patients with cancer, diabetes, pain, and more.[24]

Just because these therapies work doesn't mean we understand how they work. Many scholars argue that even if these therapies are effective, that doesn't mean we need to reinvoke concepts of vitalism to explain their effects. The mechanisms by which these therapies work could be explained by Chalmers's "easy problems," such as enhancing brain-body circuits through attention, relaxation, expectation (a part of the placebo effect), or even physical movement without needing to "go vital" or even "go spiritual."

And as long as mind-body therapies are studied only for physical health benefits such as stress reduction, depression, and brain changes, why consider alternative scientific explanations for their effects related to "loosey-goosey" terms such as *spirituality* and *vital energy*?

We can simply choose to ignore the spiritual components of the practice and not examine meditation beyond "my body, my brain, my gain." That is happening in the study of mindfulness meditation, for example.

Although it's created a booming industry for people who want to learn meditation to gain a "competitive edge," for example, in performance, scientists aren't fully examining the whole impact of mindfulness on spiritual, interpersonal, and societal development. Studies on advanced monks that report on brain changes get lots of press, but studies reporting on ordinary people's extraordinary spiritual experiences and growth while practicing meditation are largely ignored and sometimes repressed—despite data suggesting that many people have these experiences.[25]

In the mainstream scientific community, areas of study related to spiritual and energetic experiences during meditation are still considered taboo, and because of scientific gatekeeping, the impact of meditation on fostering spiritual experiences and growth (the purpose for its actual practice, from its indigenous origins) is not discussed in public. That is not only a shame—given the state of divisiveness in our world today it could be a travesty. The selective study of spirit-mind-body practices within such a narrow materialist context is certainly reflective of cultural appropriation and the dominance of Western monocultural ethnocentrism in scientific culture today—and has real costs to society.

The vitalism conundrum also arises when we study holistic therapies such as biofield or energy healing—that is, faith healing, Healing Touch, Reiki, and other related therapies. In these therapies, there is no stretching, there is no needle, and there is no directed cognitive process to try to focus attention or change breathing in any way. There is simply a person intending to heal another person through his or her connection with Divine Source and perception of movement of vital energy. It's not accomplished by using any type of physical instrument or pill whatsoever. Instead, the therapy is delivered sometimes with touch, sometimes with no touch, or even sometimes by healing from a distance.

"Antivitalism" scientists simply have skepticism about these therapies because, to date, we can't find a satisfying materialist explanation for how they work. Therefore, these scholars simply believe that these therapies are hocus pocus. When presented with well-conducted, randomized, placebo-controlled scientific studies published in high-ranking medical journals on the effects of these therapies on reducing suffering and affecting hormone function in clinical populations, these so-called skeptics have replied, "This study cannot be true because there is no such thing as energy healing."[26] Because these scientists are so attached to their particular view of the world, they cannot even fathom that these data are real because energy healing doesn't fit their model of reality.

Are the data real? Are there actually scientific data to suggest that experiences like that of two-and-a-half-year-old Meera, who experienced a complete remission from brain cancer from distance sessions by a biofield healer, could be "valid"? Can it all be explained by the placebo effect? In the next few chapters, we'll uncover the data as well as the stories from leading scientists at major universities, courageous healers willing to put their practices to the test of science, and the patients who had extraordinary experiences during these studies—all of whom have come together to unravel the mysteries of healing, learn from each other, and share the truth of what we know so far about the power and potential of human healing. Let's move forward to part II and explore the evidence.

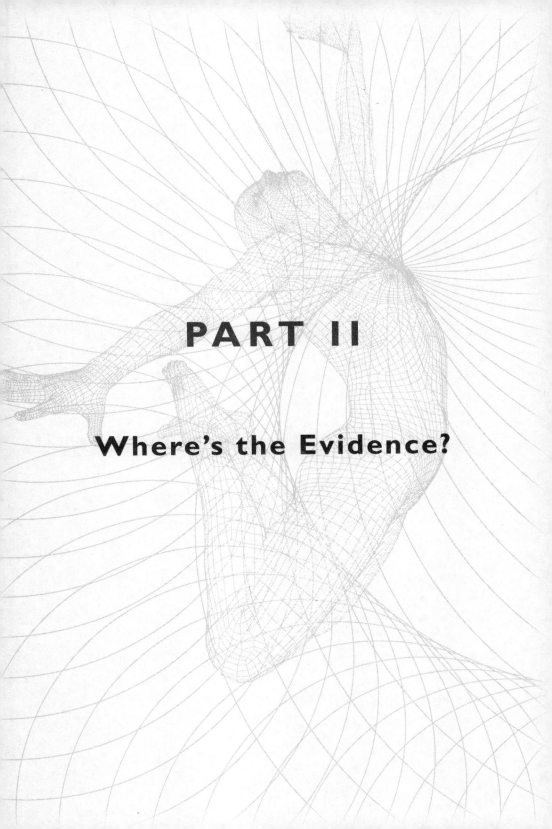

PART II

Where's the Evidence?

CHAPTER 5

Can We Heal Ourselves?
The Truth about Placebos

When we start to ask questions about the role of Consciousness and spirituality in healing, it's hard not to wonder whether it's just what scientists call the *placebo* effect.

Placebos, though well known, are perhaps the most mysterious, if not misunderstood, area of mind-body science. Although most of us have heard of placebos, we are still uncovering what the placebo effect is telling us about the power we have to heal ourselves.

To begin to understand how placebos play a role in our health and well-being and can help us foster our own healing, we need to look at both the science and the history of placebos. What's fascinating is that placebo-controlled research design came about in large part as a method to debunk energy healing!

THE MESMERIZING HISTORY OF PLACEBOS

The word *placebo* comes from the phrase "I shall please," or rather "I shall please the Lord," taken from a faulty Latin translation that dates back to the sixteenth century. Back then, so many people complained of being possessed by evil spirits that the clergy had to address the issue. To relieve anxiety in those who felt possessed, clergy began to use fake relics to "please the Lord" and their imperiled parishioners—and they seemed to work![1]

But we can really credit Franz Mesmer, an eighteenth-century physician, as the chief instigator of the popularity of the placebo-controlled trial in medicine. You might have heard of Mesmer as the father of hypnosis. What you might not have heard is that Mesmer was essentially a self-proclaimed energy healer.

Mesmer was certainly an unlikely (and often unwelcome) hero in medicine. A rebel with a cause, he was clearly dissatisfied with the medical paradigm of that time, which included the mainstream use of bleeding, purgative, and opiate therapies. He believed these therapies caused more harm than good in patients, so he sought new treatment methods that would be less damaging and equally effective.

In his search for treatments, Mesmer became aware of something he described first as *animal gravitation* and later as *animal magnetism*. He first began writing about animal gravitation in his doctoral thesis for medical school, in which he posited it was a force field that connected living things to each other and even to the planets and stars. Later, as a physician, he began focusing on the nature of this field in humans and described animal magnetism as a type of magnetic fluid. When a person had the right balance of this fluid, he believed, it led to positive health, and when the fluid was imbalanced, it led to poor health.[2]

Mesmer's initial therapeutic process involved moving magnets over a patient's body to balance the animal magnetism. He later decided the use of magnets was unnecessary, and the physician could balance a patient's field through his or her own magnetic field. This hypothesis led him to start practicing "hand passes," in which he would not touch the patient but rather pass his hands above the patient's fully clothed body as a way to both sense and alter these magnetic fields. It wasn't unlike what many biofield therapists or energy healers do today.

Later, Mesmer became convinced he didn't even need to pass his hands over a patient's body. He began to believe he possessed enough magnetic force to alter the energy of a person without having to use his hands at all. James Braid, a Scottish physician, later dubbed this technique "hypnosis."

Mesmer became famous, and in many circles infamous, for his patients' miraculous recoveries. Reports of his success in treating patients in Austria and Germany began to spread, and soon he had a long line of patients waiting to be healed by him. He set up clinics serving the rich and the poor and sought legitimacy for the science behind his clinical approach among the Viennese and Parisian scientist communities.

But Mesmer gained little support among the scientific and medical establishments, and, in fact, he soon became a liability. He displayed over-the-top showmanship around his method. His patients, often upper-class women, tended to respond dramatically to his treatments with wails and fainting. He contextualized this reaction as a "healing crisis" related to the movement of forces during the healing. Because of the dramatic show of emotion and catharsis displayed by his patients, many in the upper echelons of society found Mesmer's claims about animal magnetism and his flair for the dramatic downright distasteful. Mesmer also made what many felt were outlandish claims about the transference of his energy for healing. He claimed, for example, that he could magnetize a tree, and if patients simply touched the tree, they would recover from serious medical ailments.

In the 1800s, Isaac Newton's and Réne Descartes's *dualism* (the idea of the mind being separate from the body) heavily dominated medicine. This paradigm meant most scientists saw Mesmer as a disruptor, if not a charlatan. Mesmer gained favor in France from many, but not from King Louis XVI. The king dispatched a high-ranking scientific commission to debunk Mesmer's claims. Benjamin Franklin led the commission, which also included Antoine Lavosier and Joseph Guillotin, one of the creators of the guillotine. (Two members of the scientific commission were later beheaded with the guillotine, but that's another story.)

Members of the commission hypothesized that they could prove the patients' dramatic behaviors had no connection to Mesmer's ability or technique if they were also exposed to a "sham" situation in which they believed they were being healed by Mesmer and still had the same dramatic reaction.

The commission devised a set of experiments in which they set up sham treatments. They told patients they were being healed by Mesmer's energy directed at them, or they were touching water he had magnetized. In reality, no one was directing energy at these patients, and they were not exposed to Mesmer's magnetized water. Yet the patients responded dramatically to these sham treatments by having a healing crisis. And, in some cases, when they were exposed to the real treatment (water Mesmer had magnetized) but they weren't told of their exposure to his magnetized water, they had no reaction!

From these results, the commission concluded that Mesmer's approach was invalid and that animal magnetism did not exist.[3] Even if there was a placebo effect—meaning that so-called sham treatments could foster a healing response as a result of patients' expectations—did that mean that animal magnetism itself, or what we call the biofield, does not exist? Although many take issue with the conclusions, the experiments actually showed that the human mind is far more powerful in its effectiveness in fostering healing than we could have even imagined.

However, instead of exploring the power of the human mind to heal, the scientists at that time (and largely still at this time) thought of the mind's ability to heal as a pesky variable for which they should control in future medical studies. Thus, from the commission's studies with Mesmer, the idea of using placebos in medical science took wing. Placebo-controlled designs began to be applied to studies that examined whether specific drugs were effective in curing medical ailments beyond placebos—to determine whether the active drug, or medicine, was more powerful than the human mind's ability to heal one's self.

As we shall see in this chapter, I suggest that, based on the data, we have this model totally backward. Instead of trying to explain away the effects of placebos, we should consider the effects of placebos' fundamental healing elements—because they occur not just with Mesmer's work but with drugs for pain, depression, and even surgery. The so-called placebo effect can activate our brain-body circuitry all the way down to single-cell neurons in our brains. Let's explore what we know about placebos and what they tell us about our ability to heal ourselves.

HOW DOES A PLACEBO WORK?

Many of us have heard of placebo-controlled, randomized clinical trials (RCTs). These are research studies in which patients are randomly assigned to different groups. Patients in one group are given some active drug (thought to have some kind of specific biological action) to see what the effects are and whether the drug helps treat a disease. Patients in another group are given a placebo (a "dummy" pill that looks exactly the same but has no known chemical substance to stimulate significant biological action). People in those two groups are then compared to determine whether the active drug works by measuring its effects against those of the placebo.

If we think about how the placebo effect has been explained in modern medicine, it's really framed in a theory based on materialism. It's based on an idea that the only way to cure a disease is through taking a physical-chemical substance—the "active" treatment. Therefore, if you provide an inert ("inactive") physical substance or what is assumed to be "no active treatment," you should see no improvements.

However, scientists have now observed time and time again that a research subject who gets the inert substance, or "sham" version—the placebo—actually gets better on her or his own without any additional use of a chemically active substance!

How is this possible? How powerful is the placebo effect, and what does it tell us about the power of our own minds? Here's what we know: placebo effects occur in many treatments—for depression, pain, Parkinson's disease, and even surgery.

We might have thought placebo effects are minimal and don't matter. But in fact, studies show that placebo effects are incredibly strong for many different populations and in many settings. Following are some of the data that tell us about how powerful placebo effects are.

Placebos Account for 75 Percent of the Effects of Antidepressants on Depression

You read that right. This robust scientific finding has come not just from one study but across many studies. The scientific proof of placebo effects in depression treatments began to grab attention in 1998, when Irving Kirsch (then a professor in the Department of Psychology at the University of Connecticut and now associate director of the Harvard University Program in Placebo Studies) compiled and analyzed all the existing published results across nineteen

RCTs and 2,318 patients into a meta-analysis.[4] In these studies, he compared the effects of the antidepressants on depression in those who received placebo pills instead of the antidepressants. He found that in mild and moderate depression, the placebo effect and other "nonspecific effects" amounted to 75 percent of the reduction of the depressive symptoms. Only 25 percent of the reduction in depression could be attributed to the active drugs!

As you can imagine, this meta-analysis stirred up quite a bit of controversy among US clinicians and pharmaceutical companies. As a result, Kirsch and his colleagues then went a bit further to double-check their findings across all these studies. They got access to all the antidepressant studies collected by the Food and Drug Administration (FDA), even the ones never published in a peer reviewed journal. They found that 57 percent of the FDA trials were "failed" or "negative" trials, showing no differences between the placebo and active drug. With the FDA data, the researchers found that the placebo effect accounted for 82 percent of the drug response—even more evidence for the power of placebo effects on depression![5] The study was recently replicated again with more FDA trials, with the same result.[6]

These findings don't just stop with US studies. In the United Kingdom, for example, the National Institute for Health and Care Excellence has also reported that the differences between antidepressants and placebos are incredibly small—with only a three-point difference between placebos and active antidepressants on depression scores—considered a clinically insignificant difference.

When we take the findings of all these studies as a whole, they suggest that our minds might help to reduce our depression far more than the antidepressants we are taking. How do we continue to maximize the power of our consciousness to relieve depression—or better yet, prevent ongoing depression? Are antidepressants the answer? Antidepressant use is on the rise, and yet there are still growing rates of suffering from depression.

Given the amount of money spent on antidepressants and the residual chemicals from antidepressants in our water affecting marine life, we have to wonder whether there is a better, less toxic way of solving depression as a global health issue. The placebo discoveries with antidepressant drugs beg us to examine more closely what the placebo effect tells us about the power of our own minds. (I provide some guidelines for fostering emotional well-being in part III of this book.)

Placebo Effects Are Robust in Reducing Pain

Fabrizio Benedetti, a professor in the Department of Neuroscience at the University of Turin, Italy, and Luana Colloca, now a professor in the School of Nursing at the University of Maryland and an honorary professor at the University of Sydney, Australia, have conducted some of the most interesting and robust neuroscience research in the area of placebos and pain, or what is often called "placebo analgesia." Through carefully controlled studies, with both humans and animals, over the past few decades they and other researchers have found strong placebo effects in reducing pain.[7] How strong? A recent meta-analysis that compiled thirty-nine studies of patients who had spinal cord injuries, stroke, and multiple sclerosis found that placebo treatments (whether inert drugs or fake brain stimulation) significantly reduced central neuropathic pain in these patients, with fifteen of these studies showing changes considered clinically significant in pain levels.[8]

The effects of placebos on pain seem to get even stronger when studied in the laboratory under even more controlled conditions. A recent meta-analysis of fourteen carefully controlled experimental studies examining biological mechanisms of placebo effects on pain reported overall dramatic, substantial reductions in pain—more than six times the effectiveness in the placebo-controlled clinical trials, in which placebo groups were simply compared with drug groups.[9] In other words, the data tell us that placebos have clinically significant effects on pain.

Placebo Effects Are Significant in Surgery

The placebo effect doesn't just work for mental/emotional issues such as depression and pain. In fact, the data show that placebo responses are robust in many different contexts, including surgery. The data come from reviews of multiple studies. An initial systematic review compiled the evidence for seventy-three clinical studies that compared groups who had "real" surgery with those who had "sham" surgery. What happens in sham surgery? People randomized to the sham surgery groups never got the surgery. Instead they experienced a ritual associated with surgery and were given the expectation that they were getting the surgery and that it would help. They were presented with information, went to the hospital, received anesthesia, and in some cases were even given an incision so they thought they had had the surgery. This set up the expectation that they were going to get the surgery, and they believed they had gotten it.

In the seventy-three studies, researchers found that 74 percent (fifty-four) of those studies showed improvements in the placebo, or sham, arm. Moreover, of those fifty-four studies, 51 percent did not show a significant difference in improvement between real and sham surgery! The remaining 49 percent showed only a small difference between real and sham surgery.[10]

Recently, another research group conducted a separate meta-analysis reopening the question of the placebo effect on surgery, using more stringent criteria to review thirty-nine RCTs. Similarly, they found that overall, 65 percent of improvements from various surgical procedures could be attributed to placebo effects (see figure 5.1).[11]

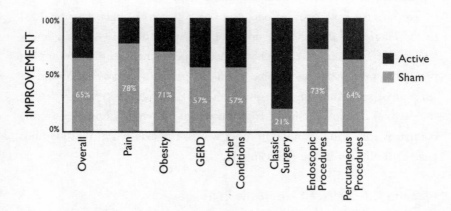

FIGURE 5.1. W. B. Jonas, C. Crawford, L. Colloca, et al., "To What Extent Are Surgery and Invasive Procedures Effective Beyond a Placebo Response? A Systematic Review with Meta-Analysis of Randomised, Sham Controlled Trials," *BMJ Open* 5, no. 12 (2015): 7, doi: 10.1136/bmjopen-2015-009655.

Placebo Effects Work, Even If We're Not "Duped"

Not only does this research call into question whether surgery or other alternatives are the best options for specific medical issues but also it might make us wonder whether being duped is the only way to get better. The cases of sham surgery are certainly dramatic. Is this type of trickery vital to fostering placebo effects? So far, initial data suggest that no, we might not have to be tricked at all.

Most of us think placebos involve some sort of fibbing or trickery. The doctors or scientists give us a sugar pill, lie, and tell us it's medicine, and we have a placebo response.

More recently, leading Harvard researchers in placebos (Irving Kirsch, Ted Kaptchuk, and colleagues) have decided to explore this question scientifically. They decided to run "open-label" placebo studies. In the first study, they randomized patients with irritable bowel syndrome (IBS) to two groups. The first group got no treatment so they could determine whether IBS symptoms would just get better on their own (we call these *natural history effects*). The second group got a placebo pill; however, this time the patients weren't tricked into thinking it was another medicine. In fact, they were told that they were getting a placebo. They were also told that research has found that placebo effects can be robust, and can lead to the reduction of symptoms (all true).

The result? Patients in the open-label placebo group got significantly better compared with those in the no-treatment group.[12] The researchers repeated the open-label placebo designs with patients with chronic low back pain and patients with migraines, again finding that openly telling patients they were getting a placebo resulted in significantly decreased pain and disability—again, without them receiving any active physical-chemical medication.[13] Similar effects have also been found now for cancer-related fatigue.[14] To further follow up on these findings, Harvard researchers are now running a large open-label placebo trial in which they plan to compare patients with IBS who are taking an open-label placebo with those on the usual double-blind placebo trial—to determine just how much it matters whether patients are told about the placebo.

For those of us taught that medicine has to be physical-chemical in nature, these results are truly mind-blowing. If patients can get better by openly being told they are getting placebos, how does that work? What neural mechanisms are at play here? Here's what else we know.

Placebo Effects Are Found Down to Our Neurons

Several studies have looked at what happens to people's brains when they receive placebos. One study conducted at the University of Michigan and published in the prestigious journal *Science* used functional magnetic resonance imaging (fMRI) to look at what happened to people's brains when they were given placebos during shock treatment.[15] First, the participants were given shocks, and the researchers examined which brain areas were activated as a result. They found typical activation of pain matrix brain areas, including the thalamus, somatosensory cortex, insula, anterior cingulate cortex (ACC), ventrolateral prefrontal cortex, and cerebellum.

Next, the patients were given a cream they were told was created to reduce the effects of the pain from shock treatment (although the cream was a placebo). This time, they found that when the participants were given this placebo cream, not only did they show increased activity in prefrontal areas of the brain before getting the shock, but they also showed decreases in activation in brain areas related to pain processing during the shock. These patients showed changes particularly in the rostral anterior cingulate cortex (rACC), which plays a role in emotion and cognition; the insula, which plays a role in the regulation of the sympathetic and parasympathetic nervous systems and the immune system; and the thalamus, which controls sensory and motor signals and regulates consciousness and alertness. Even more interesting, the decreases in brain activation in these brain areas were significantly connected to the decrease in pain people reported when getting the placebo cream.

The researchers then conducted a similar study, but this time with pain from heat versus pain from shock. They found similar results: When people anticipated getting the placebo cream, they had an increase in prefrontal cortex activity (specifically, orbitofrontal cortex and lateral prefrontal cortex) and a decrease in the same brain regions associated with pain.

Why the increase in prefrontal activity before getting the shock or the heat stimulus? It seems the participants were "readying themselves" for the pain stimulus, in part by shaping their desired expectation to have decreased pain from what was about to happen next, because of the placebo.[16] It's important to note that not all the people who got the placebo cream showed placebo responses. Some reported no decreases in pain at all even when getting the placebo cream. But for those who did, the reductions in pain processing in their brains paralleled their reports of decreased pain.

Although the brain data on the placebo cream and reduced pain is fairly mind-blowing, perhaps some of the most dramatic effects of placebos on brain function can be found in studies with people who have Parkinson's disease. Parkinson's is a disease of the nervous system that causes progressive problems with movement, sometimes called motor performance. Symptoms can include tremors, slurred speech, problems with physical balance, general stiffness, and slowing of movement. Part of the reason for these motor problems seems related to the person's inability to make dopamine in the brain, including in the basal ganglia and substantia nigra. Dopamine is a key neurotransmitter involved in emotion as well as movement. For reasons we don't understand, in patients with Parkinson's, brain cells that make dopamine die in these areas of the brain. Areas such as the striatum of the brain are also affected—if the striatum's dopamine receptors do not get enough dopamine, it affects motor performance because the striatum's lack of dopamine stimulation causes hyperactivity in the subthalamic nucleus of the brain.[17] Although there is no known cure for Parkinson's, most patients take medication to try to prevent the progression of symptoms.

Several studies have examined whether placebos might improve symptoms in patients with Parkinson's. A recent review examining placebo effects in people with Parkinson's disease reported that in sixteen of thirty-six studies, there was no difference between placebo medication and active medication on improving motor performance for patients with Parkinson's.[18] Like those who experienced pain, not all of those with Parkinson's responded to placebos, but those who did showed marked improvements. This led scientists to wonder whether those with Parkinson's who responded to placebos were showing unique brain activations. Could positive expectations of treatment affect dopamine release in these patients and therefore reduce motor symptoms such as tremors?

The Pacific Parkinson's Research Centre at Vancouver Hospital measured brain function in patients with Parkinson's via positron emission tomography

(PET) scans. The researchers reported that patients responded to placebo treatment by actually increasing their brain's own dopamine levels in the striatum—one of the brain areas we noted above, crucial for movement in patients with Parkinson's. How strong was the dopamine response? The researchers found that the increase in dopamine the patients with Parkinson's created in their own brains was comparable to the increase in dopamine they found when giving healthy volunteers methamphetamine—in other words, a substantial amount.[19] But brain responses to placebos are even more nuanced than that.

Studies have shown that placebo effects can play a significant role in deep-brain stimulation treatment for people with Parkinson's. This is a treatment in which neurons in the brain are stimulated electrically to alter the brain's circuitry in order to reduce tremors and foster better ability to move. Several studies have shown that placebo elements, particularly positive expectation, enhance the effects of deep-brain stimulation for patients with Parkinson's.[20] So scientists began to wonder whether a placebo itself might enhance the brain's circuitry in patients with Parkinson's without actually having to stimulate the brain electrically.

In a series of carefully controlled studies with patients with Parkinson's about to undergo deep-brain stimulation to help with their symptoms, Benedetti and colleagues were also able to record activity from single neural cells in the patients' brains. They found that when the patients showed a placebo response (meaning they got a placebo but thought they were getting treatment), they responded by showing not only a "clinical placebo response" of decreased rigidity of their muscles but also a "neural placebo response." Their neural firing, down to single neurons, formed a specific pattern related to their placebo response. For example, by recording responses from single neurons in the brains of the patients with Parkinson's, the researchers found a decrease in neural firing in the subthalamic nucleus—but only for those who showed a placebo response.[21] This slowing down of neural firing in the subthalamic nucleus in response to a placebo was an important finding because we know that neural firing in the subthalamic nucleus is generally overactive in patients with Parkinson's. Those who did not show a clinical placebo response (meaning that their muscle rigidity didn't change) and those who did not receive a placebo did not show these brain changes. These and similar studies demonstrate that not only do placebo responses affect us all the way to single neural cell firing but also the changes in neural firing seem to be in a beneficial direction for the patient.

Placebo Responses Don't Just Affect One Brain Pathway; They Affect Multiple Neurotransmitter Systems

Learning about these brain changes might make us wonder: Is there a specific neural pathway for placebos? It turns out there are multiple pathways, actually—and the pathways depend on what we've experienced before. The research shows that placebo responses in our bodies depend not only on our expectations of what will happen if we get a placebo but also on our conditioning, or how our body and mind respond to the placebo based on our prior experiences. For example, scientists have found that when they administered a placebo to a patient with pain, the patient's neurochemical response depended on what medications he or she was used to getting before. Our bodies make neurotransmitters that are natural painkillers, including cannabinoids and opioids—and those can help us with tolerating pain (as well as giving us natural highs). These neurotransmitter pathways are also involved when we take drugs for our pain. We can take nonsteroidal anti-inflammatory drugs (NSAIDs), which affect our natural (endogenous) cannabinoid pathway, or morphine or morphine-like drugs, which affect our endogenous opioid pathway. It seems whatever pathways we are accustomed to using are the ones that show up in placebo responses.

Specifically, placebo research has found that for patients previously given NSAIDs for their pain, when they got a placebo, their body showed activations in the body's natural (endogenous) cannabinoid pathway. However, if patients were given opioid drugs such as morphine for their pain, when they got a placebo, their bodies showed stronger activations in their natural opioid pathway. These researchers also found out that expectations of getting better, a key part of placebo response, are more associated with activating our bodies' natural opioids across the board.[22] These and other studies suggest that our responses to placebos aren't just through one pathway. When we have a placebo response, it might influence changes in many hormone and neurotransmitter pathways in the body, including our body's own opioid, cannabinoid, oxytocin, vasopressin, and dopamine systems.[23]

BREAKING DOWN PLACEBO RESPONSES: DOES PLACEBO = HEAL?

The research about depression, pain, and surgery is just the tip of the iceberg. This research, however, has shown the key elements that contribute to the placebo effect.

From this point, there is now a need for deeper research into placebos to determine the full view of how our consciousness can better foster and augment our health. The size, shape, and color of placebos, as well as the environment in which they are given, shape different responses to them.[24] Receiving placebos in a hospital, clinic, or holistic healing center affects our healing and our relationships with those helping us to heal. The way doctors and health-care providers interact with us also influences our healing path.[25] In other words, the nature and strength of our placebo effects are dependent on the context of our care as well as our mindset and relationships, and several elements foster these healing responses. This is why I propose that we reframe the term *placebo* into what I call Holistic Elements Activating Lifeforce (HEAL) for self-healing. If you don't like the term *lifeforce*, consider Holistic Elements Activating the Process of Salutogenesis (HEAPS), or self-healing.

Let's examine these aspects of HEAL: *expectations, conditioning, relationship*, and *ritual*.

Expectations refer to how much you consciously expect a treatment or medication to work. Placebo research shows that not only do we experience a more positive outcome when we expect a medicine to work, but also if we expect we are getting a medication that will harm us, we end up having a "nocebo" response—we get worse instead of better.[26] Our expectations of whether we will get better or worse play a huge role in our healing process. The medical establishment and we as patients need to set better expectations for ourselves to maximize positive outcomes and minimize negative ones to help the mind-body heal itself.

Conditioning relates to how your body-mind has experienced similar medicine before and how those previous experiences will shape the present experience with that medicine. Conditioning, a science in itself, is a powerful driver of placebo responses.[27] Generally speaking, conditioning can be considered unconscious or subconscious learning by the body-mind about the effects of a medicine as well as the setting where that treatment is received. For example, if you found before that getting a massage is relaxing, the likelihood is that your body will be ready to relax the moment you get back on a massage table, and that will help augment its healing effects.

Relationship is perhaps the least surprising, yet important, driver of placebo responses.[28] Those who have felt the emotional connection and support of a doctor, healer, therapist, or other health-care practitioner can attest to the physical and mental relief we have felt when working through a health issue. Research supports this as well: The more connected we feel with our health-care practitioners, the more likely we are to see health benefits—even down to reducing diseases such as the common cold.[29] An example of the power of a therapeutic relationship is humanistic psychologist Carl Rogers's psychotherapeutic work, not widely considered within placebo research. Rogers gave therapy sessions in which he said absolutely nothing to the patient (no advice, no formulas, no homework), and somehow this resulted in dramatic improvements in his patients. Rogers attributed this to the skill of cultivating "unconditional positive regard"—that is, a tremendous ability to provide loving presence to his patients without saying a word. We might say his unconditional positive regard was simply love in action—the strongest medicine there is. Placebo research and other related psychological fields often point to the fact that for health practitioners, not only what we do but also how we consciously show up makes a huge difference for our patients.

Ritual refers to the set and setting as well as behaviors that surround medical practices. Ritual is particularly related to meaning, which some feel is vital to the healing process and is a strong driver of placebo responses.[30] Rituals are created based on our meaning-making—for example, what the illness means to us, what it means to get better, and what actions we need to engage in to heal. Skilled health-care practitioners will understand what your illness means to you, what health means to you, and what a meaningful healing journey looks like for you. They might create, or advise you to create, your therapeutic rituals accordingly.

Indigenous cultures understand the importance of ritual in medicine. Because they do not separate medicine from spirituality, their rituals are rich with many nuances that help to foster healing responses. Native people's traditional healing rituals often involve using specific Earth elements such as feathers, herbs, and tobacco, as well as dance and song to bring Spirit into healing. These rituals set up a process to ready the body-mind to receive healing.

We forget that although we have secularized medicine in the Western world, we also engage in therapeutic ritual. Examples are doctors wearing white coats (which often contextualizes them as experts for the patients, setting up a particular power dynamic) and the standardized ways hospitals and clinics operate (patients check in at a reception desk, are ushered into a room to have their vitals checked, share their chief complaint with a nurse and then a doctor, and perhaps get a prescription). All of these rituals make a difference in the way we respond to medicine and our healing process as a result.

If we consider all the existing science behind placebos and what it tells us about the power of our consciousness to foster our own healing, it seems we need to reframe placebos better—from a model based on deception to a recognition that placebo elements are all based in consciousness. Some HEAL elements, such as expectations, are part of our conscious awareness. We might not be fully aware of other elements, such as conditioning, but they are consciousness-driven nonetheless. The more we can be aware of these HEAL elements and have them work for us, the more we can maximize our healing and the healing of others.

I believe that changing the placebo effect into the HEAL model would compel us to consider how we need to move beyond a materialist model of medicine (which assumes that physical-chemical or active treatments are the only drivers of healing effects) into a framework that honors the power of consciousness to facilitate and augment the healing process no matter what other medicines are given.

Table 5.1 summarizes the HEAL model. As you can see, the HEAL framework fits the current research data far better than the placebo model, which is based on assumptions the data suggest might not be valid.

Why am I suggesting we reframe our understanding of placebos to a consciousness-based model? In a nutshell, the eighteenth-century materialist-based premises of the placebo paradigm are outdated, and they are hindering us from understanding and using the power of our consciousness to foster healing. Let's explore these materialist myths based on the evidence we have now.

TABLE 5.1	
Placebo Model	Holistic Elements Activating Lifeforce (HEAL)
Based on materialist model (only physical/chemical substances have effects)	Based on nonmaterialist thinking (consciousness itself has effects on healing)
Contextual factors in placebos serve to "please" but not to actually "benefit" the patient. We should try to control for contextual factors that cause placebo effects in treatment studies and focus on active treatment because placebo effects are not really clinically significant.	Context is a major driver of healing effects. We should scientifically examine and maximize the effects of contextual factors such as environment, relationship, and meaning, which have been shown to foster clinically significant effects on patients, to facilitate positive healing responses.
Either active treatment (e.g., drugs or surgery) works all the time *or* it doesn't work. Elements such as expectations, conditioning, relationship, and ritual don't matter for healing. The only "real" effects of treatment must be over and above those of a placebo.	Healing can occur *both* because of an active treatment (e.g., drugs or surgery) *and* in the absence of those specific treatments through enhanced expectations, conditioning, relationship, and ritual. Enhancing these elements might even help the active treatment to be more effective.
Placebo effects are caused by a particular brain mechanism that drives healing responses.	HEAL effects are reflected in the brain. We can see the effects of healing based on our expectations and our prior experiences in the brain, but that doesn't mean the brain is causing the responses. The fact that our brains respond differently to placebos based on our prior experiences suggests that our conscious experiences are causing the brain to respond in certain ways to placebos.

Materialist Myth 1

We must always have physical medicine in order to heal ourselves; therefore placebo effects are not real.

Scientific advances in the late twentieth and early twenty-first centuries have produced significant evidence that helps us understand that our health can improve without the use of physical-chemical substances. Through the advancement of fields including psychoneuroimmunology, psychoneuroendocrinology, and systems neuroscience (all relatively new fields of study), the idea that our emotions affect our health is no longer controversial. We are now better able to track how emotions, mental states, and mind-body practices affect our physical health. This suggests that a purely materialist-based model that assumes health and disease are only influenced or cured by chemical agents is faulty. The old materialist model of placebo effects rests on the mistaken idea that healing can only be provided by use of a physical-chemical substance. It is because we (even subconsciously) subscribe to this old model that we find it so hard to believe placebo effects are real. In the newer, consciousness-based model, it's not that physical medicine never works. Drugs and surgeries can be powerful and needed treatments at times. But they are not the only means to healing and sometimes not even the most effective.

Materialist Myth 2

The placebo effect is purely psychological, meant to "please" the patients, and doesn't affect a person's healing in a significant clinical way.

The original meaning of *placebo* reflects the eighteenth-century thinking that it was to "please" but not cure the patient. That is, placebo effects were thought to appease the patient but assumed not clinically significant because they weren't chemical agents. However, the data show that placebo effects drive clinically significant improvements in health, including in surgery. As we learned, placebo responses have actually been found to alter biological states down to neural firing levels. The clinically significant data from placebo studies on depression, injuries needing surgery, pain, Parkinson's disease, and other ailments suggest that placebo effects do far more than "please" the patient—they heal.[31]

Data also suggest that rigid, either/or thinking about placebos might be outdated—that in fact it's not whether drugs or medical interventions work or whether a placebo works, but rather it's our consciousness (including our expectations to get well and our relationship with our doctor) that can modify the effectiveness of the medicine we are given. The outcome of consciousness plus medicine is not an either/or but a both/and proposition.

Materialist Myth 3

Placebo effects are caused by the brain, and there must be a single brain pathway that causes them.

The work of Benedetti and other colleagues suggests that a single brain pathway does not explain placebo responses. In fact, the data show that placebo responses are found in multiple brain pathways and in ways dependent on our prior experiences. This research suggests that placebo effects are not caused by a single mechanism in the brain, as a materialist model would suggest. Rather, our brain activity reflects our consciousness and our prior lived experience, and our conscious and unconscious conditioning is what guides our response to the medicine we are given.

SO, IS ENERGY HEALING JUST A PLACEBO?

If placebo effects are found during surgery, why wouldn't they be found in energy healing? Indeed, placebo effects have been found in all types of placebo-controlled trials—including studies of integrative health treatments such as acupuncture and energy healing as well as drugs and surgery.[32] The million-dollar question when it comes to understanding the effects of energy healing is this: Is there something to working with the biofield that takes healing above and beyond placebo effects? Some might say it more bluntly: Is energy real?

In chapters 7 and 8 of this book, focused on the question of whether we can heal each other with biofield therapies, I'll share what RCTs—with animals, cells, and humans—actually tell us about the effects of energy and biofield healing beyond placebo elements—and what that means for how we can heal others. But before we go there, let's look at even more data that explore whether, and how, we can heal ourselves with mind-body-spirit practices.

CHAPTER 6

Can We Heal Ourselves?
Mind-Body Therapies

Not too long ago, I gave a talk at a business conference in which I shared with the attendees how the runaway train of our "sick-care" system (which should be a health-care system) was costing society billions of lives and trillions of dollars. In the talk, I suggested that the more we invest in providing these evidence-based self-care approaches, the more we can prevent disease, reduce suffering, and foster flourishing in society. The talk was well received, but I felt the real impact of the talk about eight months afterward, when serendipitously talking with one of the attendees, William W. Brown. Brown, a businessman in his seventies, is well respected as a community and philanthropic leader. He founded Legacy Early College, the largest Title I charter school for underprivileged youth in South Carolina, which ensures that every student receives a stellar education and opportunities to attend college regardless of income. While I was visiting my parents, Brown, who lived in the same town, invited my husband and me to dine with him. "I just want to tell you," Brown said to me over a casual lunch, "your talk changed my life."

I was thrilled to hear this and inquired exactly what he meant. "We hear about trends like yoga and meditation, and of course we all know there's a huge boom in the wellness industry. But until I saw the data you presented,

I never actually realized that I could heal myself. I never realized I had that much power over my own health."

He explained that since he had heard my talk, he felt motivated to take charge of his health. He no longer felt afraid of or even bought into everything he had been told about aging and the possibilities of medical illnesses he might get as a result of the aging process. Instead of feeling helpless, he now felt empowered to jump-start his own healing. He committed to meditating every day. He changed his diet to a vegan diet, engaged in regular exercise, and realized how honing his expectations and intentions for healing—key areas on which I provide guidance in part III of this book—could augment the results he wanted to see. As a result, eight months after my talk, he felt healthier and more empowered than he had ever felt before and remained, happily, free of diabetes, heart disease, and other so-called aging-related diseases. Brown was a living example of preventative medicine, empowered by the knowledge of his own healing power.

Brown also recognized that the profound peace he was feeling from his regular meditation practice would benefit underprivileged students. Even though his charter school was successful in sending students to college, these students often faced significant stress from coming into a completely different environment—which often drove them to anxiety, depression, and sometimes dropping out of college. He decided to implement a schoolwide mindfulness program that would benefit students, staff, and teachers by creating a mindful school culture and providing "tools for life."

"More than anything," he shared, "I now realize that I have more control over my health than I thought ever possible, and I realize that every child deserves the peace that I get from my practice."

What do we really know about these mind-body practices in terms of their ability to foster healing? In this chapter, I focus primarily on a few ancient practices gaining global popularity. We are seeing more of them integrated into clinics, hospitals, and schools than ever before. We'll examine the data behind mind-body therapies through systematic reviews and meta-analyses that compile and analyze numbers of clinical research studies, including randomized controlled trials (RCTs)—still considered the "gold standard" of study design in medical research.

We'll also explore how the science of psychoneuroimmunology (PNI), and particularly the role of the vagus nerve, is helping us understand how these mind-body self-care practices get under the skin and provide physical as well as emotional and mental health benefits. We'll explore how the vagus nerve helps integrate both the top-down (mind) aspects of how these mind-body practices work and the bottom-up (body) mechanisms that foster mind-body healing effects.

In addition, we'll explore areas of these mind-body approaches not generally discussed in the Western science and health-care worlds—specifically, what these practices have shared about the spiritual and energetic aspects of healing. Beyond the physical mechanisms of healing, what do we know about how ancient cultures described the healing process that occurs with mind-body therapies? The ancients talked about biofield concepts such as life force, prana, and qi as playing a central role in these mind-body therapies. Does this so-called vital life force, part of what we scientists now currently call the *biofield*, really have anything to do with healing ourselves? Let's start with yoga.

YOGA: ANCIENT PRACTICES, NEW UNDERSTANDINGS

Yoga, as you might know, is not simply an excuse to buy Lululemon pants! This spirit-mind-body system is thousands of years old. The meaning of the Sanskrit word *yoga* is "union," or "to yoke." It quite simply unifies our "little c" consciousness with "big C" Consciousness. Put another way, yoga is a path to reunite ourselves with our soul, spirit, or God-consciousness, however we describe it. Different sages have described yoga in different terms, but all describe the path of yoga as a method of leading us to the "big C" Consciousness I described in chapter 3—unbounded, blissful, and ever-knowing Consciousness. For example, yoga sage Patanjali, whose eight-limbed path of yoga is a foundation for practice today, wrote in his Yoga Sutras sometime around the second century BCE, "*Yoga chitta vritti nirodha*," which basically means, "Yoga is the cessation of the fluctuations of the mind."[1] By ceasing the fluctuations of the mind, we can access the deeper aspects of God-consciousness, which expand beyond our emotional, mental, and social conditioning. Other yoga sages, such as Vyasa, describe the path of yoga as leading to bliss, an aspect of unbounded Consciousness. In the first line of his commentary on Patanjali's Yoga Sutras, Vyasa states, "Yoga samadhi"— meaning, essentially, yoga is a path to blissful union.[2]

Although yoga originated in India, it is said and understood to belong to no one religion, no one country, and no one school of thought. Despite what some modern-day teachers and businesses might have you believe with their trademarks—no one "owns" yoga. The most adept yoga practitioners and teachers have emphasized that yoga is simply a systematic process to guide one toward self-realization, peace, and spiritual liberation. In fact, insights and practices from yogic teachings have been compared with other spiritual and religious traditions, including Christianity.[3]

What is this systematic process? We might think it is simply a series of poses we use to stretch our bodies in certain ways. But actually, the asanas, or physical postures, are just one part of a whole system Patanjali highlighted in his Yoga Sutras, and they are considered foundational to classical yoga practice.

Patanjali described an *ashtanga* ("eightfold") sequential path of yoga that is basically a guide for living a full human life:

The first foundational step is *yama*, creating and living by a code of ethics (in yoga, this code consists of nonviolence, nonstealing, truthfulness, nonpossessiveness, and sexual fidelity or restraint).

The second step is *niyama*, which encourages us to create disciplined habits to better carry out those codes of ethics to better align our body-mind with Truth.

The third step is *asanas*, or the physical postures that we are familiar with in the West from yoga classes. These are supportive physical postures to help foster and balance flowing currents of energy in our bodies. Cultivating this harmonious flow of energy in the body allows the mind to obtain greater stillness and less disturbance. Practicing the yoga asanas is actually meant to ready the body for meditation or prayer.

The fourth step, *pranayama*, involves specific breathwork practices to allow us to further direct and balance *prana*, or life force energy, in our bodies—again, with the intention of settling the mind for meditative and prayerful practice.

The fifth step, *pratayahara*, is to temporarily withdraw from the outside world and our attachment to sensory stimuli and go inward to better access deeper levels of knowing. This helps keep us from expending all our energy outward, in a "doing loop" of life, so that we can better open to inner guidance.

The sixth step, *dharana*, is the process of cultivating concentration by focusing our consciousness in a single-pointed direction—which could be the breath, a word, or another point of focus—in order to train the mind.

The seventh step, *dhyana*, is the practice of broader awareness meditation, in which we move beyond single-pointed concentration into a more open, moment-to-moment awareness.

Successfully embarking upon and mastering these seven steps leads us to the eighth and ultimate step, *samadhi*, the realization of God-consciousness characterized by its qualities of *sat-chit-ananda*, or blissful, omniscient, unbounded Consciousness.

Through Patanjali's eightfold yoga path, we can see how behavioral self-assessment and modifications (the yama and niyama of ethics and discipline), along with physical practices, awareness, mastery of life energy (the asanas, pranayama), and dharana and dhyana (meditation), or ability to cultivate both concentration and moment-to-moment awareness beyond the conditioned self—all come together to foster a realized life. Yoga is therefore a prescribed path of growth that ultimately leads to spiritual freedom.

However, in the West yoga is rarely scientifically studied as it was meant to be practiced—as a whole system of self-care that incorporates breathwork, concentration, discipline, ethics, meditation, physical postures, and sensory withdrawal for spiritual development. Western science leans toward reductionism (looking at things in parts instead of as a whole) and is generally loathe to study anything that would seem "religious" or "spiritual," particularly from a "foreign" culture. Scientists and those that fund them, therefore, decided to study certain aspects of meditation and yoga over others, more for symptom reduction than self-realization. In the West, we've studied bits and pieces of yoga, such as specific yoga asanas, or sets of postures; specific pranayama practices, or breathwork exercises; and a few mantra meditation and prayer practices as standalone tools for health.

As a consequence, similar to the study of many holistic approaches and therapies, Western research on meditation and yoga is limited by the domination of ethnocentrism, materialism, and reductionism in science and medicine.

Does that mean these yoga studies are not legitimate? Absolutely not. In fact, in Ayurveda, an ancient, whole-systems medical practice from India, specific yoga breathwork exercises and physical postures are often prescribed for specific ailments, so it makes sense to study these pieces, particularly if we are targeting a specific clinical condition. Although our knowledge of yoga as a system to foster self-realization is largely incomplete, we are learning more and more about specific yoga practices to help alleviate certain types of suffering. Most of these studies have been done with breathwork as well as yoga asanas, or physical postures. Several systematic reviews of the studies and meta-analyses have been conducted regarding yoga in the past decade. There are many different forms of yoga practice, mostly examining asana practice or training in the physical postures, that have been studied scientifically. What do the studies on yoga asana as a whole tell us so far?

Yoga reduces pain. A meta-analysis incorporating sixteen studies with 1,007 patients who presented with back pain, carpal tunnel, headache/migraine, irritable bowel syndrome (IBS), muscle soreness, labor pain, or rheumatoid arthritis reported that overall, yoga reduced disability and pain and had positive effects on mood.[4] Similar results have been released by the Agency for Healthcare Research and Quality (AHRQ), which reports that yoga has small to moderate but significant effects on chronic pain and function.

The agency notes that more high-quality studies are needed to deeply investigate the effects of yoga on pain.[5]

Yoga reduces depression and fatigue in cancer survivors. The most recent meta-analysis of twenty-nine randomized controlled trials (RCTs) in 1,828 cancer survivors found significant, moderate effects on reducing depression and significant but small effects on reducing fatigue, but no statistically significant effects on changing self-reported quality of life. Overall, session length mattered—the longer the sessions were, the greater the effects seemed to be on depression.[6]

Yoga decreases fatigue in patients with multiple sclerosis (MS). A recent meta-analysis of ten RCTs in 693 patients with MS determined that yoga decreased their fatigue compared with the usual care for patients with MS, with effects no different from those of exercise. As in the analysis of patients with cancer, yoga didn't seem to affect their self-reported quality of life.[7]

Yoga reduces headaches. A recent meta-analysis of five RCTs reported that yoga decreases headache duration, frequency, and intensity of pain. Importantly, these effects seemed to work for tension-type headaches, not migraines.[8]

Yoga reduces menopausal symptoms. A meta-analysis of thirteen RCTs with 1,306 patients determined that compared with usual care, yoga reduces menopausal symptoms—including psychological symptoms (such as depression and irritability), urogenital symptoms (such as trouble retaining urine), and vasomotor symptoms (such as night sweats and hot flashes). When compared with exercise interventions, yoga worked about the same as exercise in reducing menopausal symptoms, except for reducing vasomotor symptoms, in which yoga seemed to have an advantage.[9]

Yoga might help with some aspects of mental health. Several reviews have examined the effects of yoga on adult patients with major depressive disorder and suggest that yoga might have some positive effects for their depressed mood.[10] A few studies suggest that yoga can be helpful as an adjunctive (additional) therapy for children with attention-deficit/hyperactivity disorder (ADHD) and patients with schizophrenia. The data are limited as to whether yoga has any effect on anxiety.[11] Similarly as with pain, the consensus is that studies with larger numbers of patients are needed to draw firm conclusions on how helpful yoga can be for mental ailments.

WHAT ABOUT BREATHING?

Another key aspect of yoga, as we explored above, is pranayama, or working with the breath to move vital energy throughout the body. The Sanskrit term *pranayama* actually means "life force extension," with *prana* referring to *life force* and *ayama* referring to *extension* or *expansion*. Pranayama practices involve directing the breath to certain parts of the body, often with timed breathing and specific breathing rhythms.

There are not as many studies on specific pranayama exercises as there are on yoga asanas, and in general there should be more rigorous studies that have sufficient controls with which to compare the pranayama breathing practices. However, the studies that do exist report that pranayama exercises, such as *bhramari* pranayama and *bhastrika* pranayama, increase the function of the "rest-and-digest" part of the body's nervous system known as the parasympathetic nervous system. These studies found that these pranayama practices lowered blood pressure and heart rate.[12] A recent systematic review of studies on breathing techniques for chronic obstructive pulmonary disease (COPD) reported that timed breathing pranayama exercises significantly increased the walking capacity and quality of life of patients with COPD.[13]

As with current comparisons between yoga and exercise, in which yoga is generally found equal to exercise in reducing symptoms, current studies show that pranayama and other types of breathing exercises work for enhancing parasympathetic nervous system activity. Currently in the West, secularized breathing techniques that stem from pranayama and related Tibetan practices (e.g., Tummo) are becoming popular—such as the Wim Hof method, for example.[14]

What we can conclude from the limited research on pranayama and related breathing techniques is that these approaches all appear to have meaningful and sometimes profound effects on the nervous system, and that much more should be explored to better understand the impact of these breathing methods on our longer-term emotional, mental, and physical health.

MEDITATION: DIFFERENT PATHWAYS, SIMILAR DESTINATION

As we explored earlier in this chapter, meditation is actually considered part of the path of yoga. However, as with breathwork techniques, meditation practices are quite diverse, with many different forms not only in India but also in many cultures and spiritual traditions, including Buddhism, Christianity, Hinduism, Islam, Jainism, Judaism, and others.[15] At least 15 million Americans report that they engage in regular sitting meditation, whether it be described as mantra, mindfulness, or spiritual meditation.[16] This doesn't even count movement-based meditations such as qigong/chi gong and tai chi that other people in the United States report practicing.[17]

What exactly is meditation, and what distinguishes it from prayer? The answer depends on who you ask. Let's dive into a few types of meditation practices, including the data behind their health effects, to explore how we can work with them to cultivate greater health and well-being.

Mindfulness Meditation

Currently in the West, mindfulness meditation has become popular. Corporate interest in the practice has grown into a multi-billion-dollar industry—not without concern or critique.[18] Mindfulness meditation, as it is called in the West, has been largely drawn from Buddhist *Vipassana* ("insight") meditation. It is described as the cultivation of "nonjudgmental, moment-to-moment awareness." Initially during this type of meditation, a practitioner might choose to focus her or his awareness on the breath, body sensations, or even a more broad, "open" awareness, depending on the training.[19] By attending to what is here in the present moment, mindfulness helps us to train the mind to observe emotions, sensations, and thoughts without becoming attached to them or pushing them away.

This practice has roots in deep philosophy on the nature and process of accessing full Consciousness, as we explored in chapter 3. In the West, mindfulness meditation as it is taught in programs such as mindfulness-based stress reduction (MBSR) often first involves learning to pay attention to our natural breathing and experiencing the breath moment to moment while letting sensations and thoughts come and go. Such programs also teach body scanning, a method of paying attention to bodily sensations, starting with the feet and scanning all the way up to the head, along with paying attention to the breath while letting thoughts come and go. These practices are all rooted in the Vipassana tradition.

Vipassana meditation practitioners might explain mindfulness practice like this: Humans live most of our lives in a cycle of attachment and avoidance (I like this/"yum"; I dislike that/"yuck"). Because we are constantly pulled into this yum/yuck thinking, we actually have habits that create causal chains of reaction and conditioning. Through mindfulness practice, including meditation, we learn how to simply be in the moment and observe the flow of yum/yuck thinking, including our impulses and reactions. As a result, we learn how to cultivate the stillness of observation in a dynamic world, recognizing the impermanence of situations and things, experiencing them fully for what they are but not getting attached to them or pushing them away when they come and go. Ancient traditions held that when we open our minds to deeper awareness by ceasing to engage in the causal chains of attachment and aversion, we can better recognize the ever-present, full Consciousness and, eventually, become self-realized, or spiritually liberated.[20] Mindfulness meditation practices were thus created as a pathway toward self-realization.

MINDFULNESS FOR HEALTH:
WHAT THE RESEARCH SAYS

Of course, because we tend to live in a material world, as with studies on yoga, empirical research on mindfulness meditation has been more focused on symptom reduction, not self-realization. One might wonder whether the scientists have it backward: Wouldn't exploring how mindfulness affects the process of self-realization actually lead us to better understand its resultant effects on symptom reduction? Instead, mindfulness meditation is often advertised in the West as some type of mind-body pill we take to reduce our discomfort, as if that were the point of the practice. Still, given the high prevalence of chronic mental and physical disorders in society today, exploring whether mindfulness practices can aid in mental and physical health is an important and legitimate area for current scientific discovery. Beyond the commercial hype, what do we really know about the health effects of mindfulness meditation practice?

Mindfulness meditation programs help reduce the experience of pain. A recent meta-analysis examined thirty-eight RCTs of mindfulness meditation by 3,526 patients with fibromyalgia, headache, IBS, osteoarthritis, and other conditions, and determined that mindfulness had small but significant effects on reducing chronic pain and depression as well as improving quality of life.[21]

Mindfulness meditation programs seem helpful for mental health. Another recent meta-analysis of forty-seven studies of mindfulness meditation by 3,515 participants suggested it is effective in reducing anxiety and depression, but with effects no different than those of exercise or behavioral therapies. However, mindfulness meditation did not appear to meaningfully change eating behaviors, sleep, weight, or mood.[22] Another systematic review of twenty-four studies reported that mindfulness-based interventions for employees were helpful overall in reducing their anxiety, depression, distress, and emotional exhaustion, as well as improving their sense of personal accomplishment and self-compassion.[23]

Mindfulness meditation programs help reduce emotional suffering in cancer patients. A systematic review of twenty-two studies reported significant effects of mindfulness-based interventions on anxiety and depression in 1,403 adult patients with cancer.[24]

Mindfulness meditation training affects us down to our neurons and immune cells. Several studies have found brain changes occurring with mindfulness training in novices (those who don't have a history of meditating). Those studies have found changes in brain structure and function that occur after mindfulness training, such as changes in gray matter density in the hippocampus (an area related to memory), reduced activity of the amygdala (an area related to emotional reactivity), and decreased "default mode network" activity across brain regions (areas related to self-referential thinking and mind wandering). As we might suspect, these brain changes also effect changes in participants' abilities to regulate attention and emotions.[25] In terms of mindfulness meditation training's effects on immune system function, a recent review of twenty RCTs on mindfulness training of 1,602 patients suggested that the results of these studies show some consistency in reducing C-reactive protein (CRP, a protein associated with inflammation), decreasing cellular transcription factor NF-kB (which also helps regulate inflammation), and increasing telomerase activity (which helps to prevent cellular aging).[26] However, it's unclear whether these immune effects are specific to mindfulness training practice or could result from other types of mind-body practices, and it's unclear how long these changes might last.

Is mindfulness meditation *just* relaxation? Do we know whether these mindfulness meditation trainings are actually successful in bringing people to a greater state of mindfulness? Is there something unique about mindfulness-based interventions that actually drives these health effects, or are the improvements all caused by other factors, such as relaxation and social support?

To help answer this question, in the early 2000s as a graduate student at the University of Arizona, I conducted my first RCT to find out whether mindfulness meditation was effective in reducing mental and emotional distress and improving mood states in stressed medical and premedical students. I was curious about whether the effects of mindfulness meditation could be explained simply by relaxation, by slowing breathing, or by some other means. I compared a group of students receiving mindfulness meditation training with a group of students getting comprehensive relaxation training (the relaxation comparison group) and a group of students receiving no training at all (the control group). Shockingly, this study, published in 2007 in *Annals of*

Behavioral Medicine, was the first RCT that compared mindfulness meditation training with another active treatment to find out whether there were any unique effects of mindfulness over and above relaxation.

Stress and burnout in medical and premedical students is problematic and often can lead to continued problems even after graduation, including suicidal thoughts.[27] However, at that time, not many researchers were addressing how these students could reduce their stress and learn tools they could use in their personal lives and perhaps even their medical practices. When I put out the call for medical and premedical students to engage in this stress-management study, I had a long list of eager volunteers.

Students in the mindfulness meditation intervention received MBSR, a standardized treatment that includes sitting meditation, yoga, and body scanning, as well as class discussion. We also added lovingkindness meditation, in which students were taught to send lovingkindness to themselves and others. Students in the relaxation group received tried and true, evidence-based relaxation training including progressive muscle relaxation (in which one tenses and then relaxes muscles), autogenic training (in which one uses a type of verbal suggestion to relax the body, such as "my legs feel heavy"), and diaphragmatic breathing training. Both groups were treated by highly trained professionals who had years of experience teaching the techniques. I compared students in these two active-treatment groups with a waitlist control group of students who just went on with their lives as usual and didn't attempt any additional type of mind-body practice.

Having had experience with meditation and an understanding of mindfulness, I suspected that a key ingredient for mindfulness meditation interventions was the training, which helped keep one's attention on the present moment and therefore helped one be less likely to engage in ruminative thinking. Rumination, often referred to as "chewing one's cud," is the process of thinking about something over and over to the point of being stuck in a loop of unhelpful thinking. Although human minds have this natural tendency, a significant number of people with anxiety, depression, and stress engage in high amounts of ruminative thinking, meaning they keep rehearsing the same thoughts in their head—which often drives them to feel more anxious and depressed.[28] Ruminative thoughts tend to pull people into the past ("Why did he/she/I do/say that?") or the future ("What will happen if he/she/I do. . .")—therefore keeping them from the magic of the present moment. Might mindfulness meditation reduce distress, at least in part, by reducing the tendency to rehash troubling thoughts about the past or the future and help us stay in the present moment?

Indeed, what I found was that mindfulness meditation was unique in its ability to reduce ruminative thinking, and that decrease in rumination in turn reduced distress. Mindfulness meditation practice, not relaxation techniques, helped people to get out of the circular thinking, and disengaging from this loop helped reduce the anxiety and depression for the students in that group. This result suggested, indeed, a unique potential added value of mindfulness meditation over straight relaxation practice—an ability to get out of circular rumination by staying in the present moment, allowing one's thoughts to come and go without getting looped into them.

Concentrative Meditation

Mindfulness processes differ from practices called *concentrative* meditation techniques, in which the intention is not to foster a greater capacity for broad attention but to focus our awareness more specifically to help quiet and focus the mind. The overarching understanding is this: By quieting and focusing the mind on a particular object of reverence, we develop a silence that allows us to better connect with Consciousness (or Divinity). Our attention can be placed, for example, on a holy word, an energy center, or even on nature to help cultivate this quieting of the mind and orientation toward the Divine.

The processes and practices of concentrative meditation, as understood by Western scientists, are extensive and encompass many traditions, including centering prayer in Christian traditions, chakra-based and mantra-based meditations in several East and South Asian traditions, Dadirri' practices in Australian aboriginal culture, and more.[29] However, all these practices are described as means for bringing ourselves closer to experiencing Divine presence. In Christian centering prayer, one cultivates interior silence as a means to experience the presence of God. Often, a word is used to focus attention on God's presence.[30] Similarly, in Dadirri' practice, one cultivates inner silence as a means of listening deeply to nature to bring forth quiet, still awareness.

In some traditions, concentrative and mindfulness practices are synergistic. For example, in the Vipassana tradition, narrowing the concentrative focus onto a singular object (as in the *anapana sati* meditation, in which the concentration is on the breath coming in and out of the nose and body) is almost considered a prerequisite for engaging the mind in broader moment-to-moment awareness anchored in bodily sensation.[31] And, as I discussed earlier, in Patanjali's eightfold yogic path, the last three steps are dharana, dhyana, and samadhi. He described a pathway whereby one develops concentrated focus (dharana), which helps the mind to better engage in broader, open awareness devoid of attachment and aversion (dhyana), leading ultimately to merging with Consciousness (samadhi). Tibetan Buddhist teachers have also often declared that both concentrative (sometimes also called *focused awareness*) practices and mindfulness (sometimes called *open awareness*) practices are fundamental to the experience of full meditative states.[32]

Concentrative practices have also been described as having stages. In Buddhist meditation theory, which informs, for example, *bhavana metta*, or lovingkindness practices, successive levels of concentration bring the practitioner from the beginnings of being able to focus attention in a single direction to essentially merging with that object of attention so that there is no sense of separation between the observer and observed—leading, ultimately, to the state of oneness with Consciousness.[33] The ability to focus attention becomes more effortless and the experience more transcendent with continued practice and time.

Thus we can see that although the practices in concentrative meditation techniques are global and vast in diversity, all have a common purpose not unlike the original purpose of mindfulness meditation: to bring us into a greater, whole Consciousness. How the meditation traditions describe that Consciousness is dependent on the cultures in which they originated.

We can consider all of these concentrative meditation practices different pathways to the same destination. But how effective are they for mental and physical health? The real answer is that we haven't conducted enough deep study on all the varieties of concentrative meditation and contemplation practices to know. Many studies have been conducted on a practice called transcendental meditation (TM), but only a handful of studies focus on different mantra meditation practices, such as Buddhist *shamatha* practice, mantra repetition, and others. There is little research on the effects of centering prayer and virtually no studies on indigenous forms of concentrative and contemplative meditation practice.

Given the limited research at present, what do we know about the power of these practices for self-healing? Following is the most robust finding so far, based on systematic reviews of many research studies.

Concentrative meditation positively affects our cardiovascular system. Although there have not been as many recent neuroimaging and physiology studies with concentrative meditation techniques as there have been with mindfulness meditation, several studies, including those conducted decades ago, have indicated that TM reduces blood pressure at clinically significant levels.[34] However, several investigators noted that further studies should be conducted with active control groups, in which meditation could be compared, for example, with relaxation or exercise.[35] The positive effects of concentrative meditation practices on heart health might not involve mantras only: One study compared rosary prayer with mantra meditation and found that both practices can slow down breathing and improve heart functioning.[36]

Although mindfulness and concentrative meditation practices are considered sitting practices, beyond yoga what do we know about movement-based meditative practices—particularly those said to incorporate the biofield, or sensing and moving subtle energy, in their practice?

Movement-Based Meditation: The Flow of Health Benefits from Qigong and Tai Chi

Although ancient teachings on sitting meditation and yoga clearly described aspects of the practices related to working with the biofield (specifically, prana) for fostering health, perhaps the movement-based meditation practices such as qigong (also called *chi gong* and *chi kung*) and one of its forms, a martial art called *tai chi*, were most explicit about the fundamental role of subtle energy in fostering health and healing. The term *qigong* itself is often translated as "energy work." Qigong is considered more modern terminology for an ancient set of practices. At least thirty names were used for these practices in ancient times. In fact, it wasn't until the 1950s that the Chinese government accepted the name *qigong* to describe these sets of practices.[37]

Early records of the actual term *qigong* appear in texts from the Ming Dynasty (1368–1644). Accounts of it as a spiritual self-healing practice date all the way back to the sixth century BCE, with Taoist traditions describing it as *dao-yin* ("leading and guiding the energy"), *yang sheng* ("nourishing and guiding the forces of life"), and *tu gu na xin* ("expelling the old energy; drawing in the new"), to name a few. The classic second-century text *Yi Jing* ("Book of Changes") describes the relationship of qi with humans, heaven, and Earth, and is considered foundational for qigong. In the classic Taoist text *Dao De Jing*, qi and its relationship to mind and Consciousness is described eloquently by Zhuang Zi (famous Taoist practitioner and disciple of the "father of Taoism," Lao Zi):

> Unify your will and don't listen with your ears, but with your
> mind. No, don't listen with your mind, but listen with your *qi*.
> Listening stops with the ears, the mind stops with perception,
> but qi is empty and waits on all things. Tao gathers in emptiness
> alone. Emptiness is the fasting of the mind.[38]

What was Zhaung Zi, who was known to highlight the spiritual aspects of qi in his teachings, saying? Qi is not just defined shallowly as "life energy." Qi is also considered pure potentiality—the part of the formless that can, may, and does take form. This is similar to the concept of Shakti in Tantric traditions: Shakti is considered the energetic power behind the manifest universe.[39]

Like texts in meditation and yoga, teachings on these ancient practices reveal the fundamental importance of qi in leading us to a deeper understanding of Consciousness. The spiritual meanings of qi are vast and deep and, for most of us, likely require a lifetime of contemplation to fully comprehend. However, the ancient traditions clearly described through texts and oral history the relationship between qi, or life energy, and self-healing and health—and how each of us can access this practice now, for our own health, well-being, and growth. As with yoga, qigong describes intentional use of the breath and movement for enhanced health and longevity. For example, Zhaung Zi describes in the *Dao De Jing*:

> *Exhaling through the mouth while exercising the breath,*
>
> *Spitting out the old breaths while drawing in the new,*

Moving like the bear, stretching like a bird,

This is simply the art of longevity!

And the aim of those scholars who practice dao-yin.[40]

Because dao-yin and, later, qigong practices were described as promoting health, they were often recognized over millennia as powerful methods for cultivating bodily strength and longevity.

QIGONG AND TAI CHI FOR HEALTH: WHAT THE RESEARCH SAYS

Currently, qigong is categorized for different purposes: There is medical qigong, a self-care practice we use to promote our own health (this form appears to be the modern version of Taoist dao-yin practices); there is external qigong, in which a learned practitioner can use qi to foster healing in another person; and there is martial arts qigong, in which martial artists can use specific qigong practices for self-defense purposes. Medical qigong practices were widely used in the Ming and Ching Dynasties (1368–1911) for health, and currently in the West as well as in China there is a resurgence of the study and practice of qigong for health and longevity. In addition, a martial art form known as tai chi has gained popularity in the West. It is said that tai chi (also known as *ta ji quan*) borrowed exercises from qigong martial arts practices, but it is also used as a self-care practice for cultivating health and wellness.[41] What do we know about the health benefits of medical qigong and tai chi?

Qigong and tai chi reduce blood pressure. A systematic review of twenty-one studies with 1,604 patients with hypertension, diabetes, obesity, and metabolic syndrome reported that qigong and tai chi produce a small but significant reduction in blood pressure (both systolic and diastolic) compared with no treatment. In addition, body mass index (BMI) was also significantly reduced even when qigong and tai chi were compared with exercise.[42]

Qigong and tai chi improve functioning in those with chronic disease. A recent systematic review of forty-seven studies examined the effects of tai chi for conditions including arthritis, osteoarthritis, hypertension, and more. They found that those patients training in tai chi showed significantly improved movement performance (including balance and gait) and cardiovascular fitness across these conditions.[43] Another recent meta-analysis of twenty-one studies, including fifteen RCTs in 735 patients with Parkinson's disease, found that these practices improved motor functioning (including fall risk) as well as reduced depression and improved quality of life.[44]

Qigong and tai chi help cancer patients with sleep and fatigue. A recent updated meta-analysis that included twelve clinical trials with qigong and tai chi since 2014 suggested these therapies are helpful in improving sleep quality and reducing fatigue in patients with cancer.[45] Another systematic review examining six RCTs of tai chi in 373 patients found similar effects, reporting that tai chi reduced short-term cancer-related fatigue significantly more than exercise or psychological support did, with longer interventions having greater effect.[46] The effects of qigong and tai chi on mental health and quality of life in patients with cancer were more mixed—with some systematic reviews reporting small effects and some reporting none.[47]

Qigong and tai chi improve immunity. A systematic review of sixteen studies (including seven RCTs) found that people who practiced tai chi had improvements in cell-mediated immunity as well as antibody responses.[48] Another systematic review of eight RCTs found that practicing tai chi improved lipid profiles (i.e., high-density and low-density lipoproteins) in a variety of patients, including those with cardiovascular disease, hypertension, and diabetes.[49] Similar findings have been reported in other systematic reviews examining the effects of these therapies on immune function, with a recent meta-analysis pointing to positive effects of qigong and tai chi on reducing inflammation as measured by inflammatory proteins C-reactive protein and interleukin-6.[50]

COMMON PATHWAYS FOR HEALING OURSELVES THROUGH MIND-BODY PRACTICES

After reading this chapter, you might have noticed that the data from studies of these different mind-body therapies are somewhat similar in terms of showing positive effects on reducing blood pressure, improving immunity, affecting brain function, and reducing mental and physical symptoms of disease.

You might also have noticed that the underlying philosophies of practices including concentrative meditation, mindfulness meditation, qigong, tai chi, and yoga are really more similar than different. Their philosophical and practice-related commonality is a universal Consciousness beyond our cultural and social conditioning (sometimes described as Oneness, Emptiness, or God).

The path toward healing is to connect with this larger Consciousness in order to fully realize our potential as human beings. Healing is a spiritual as well as emotional and physical process.

All of these practices describe a vital life force (sometimes called *qi*, *chi*, *prana*, or other terms) that links our bodies and minds to the experience of Consciousness. We can connect with this vital life force and direct it for healing through breathwork, movement, focusing the mind, and broadening our attention. These practices foster healing by restoring harmony between us and our environment and promote longevity. In addition to these commonalities in philosophy and practice, we also see commonalities in how meditation, tai chi, yoga, and similar practices affect the body, including improving immunity and cardiovascular function. Why is that? Is there a common mechanism that explains their effects?

HOW MIND-BODY HEALING WORKS: THE ROLE OF THE "WANDERER"

Recall that several decades ago we didn't even believe that the brain and body were connected. Now, thanks to fields such as psychoneuroimmunology and the hard work and collaboration between immunologists, endocrinologists, psychologists, and neuroscientists, we are beginning to understand just how connected our minds and bodies are—including how our bodily signals influence our brain (not just how the brain influences the body). A key player in understanding the mind-body link and how these mind-body practices affect healing is the vagus nerve. The Latin term *vagus* means "wandering" or "straying." It's the biggest cranial nerve in our body, and it wanders from the brain all around the body to connect with many different organs.

The vagus is basically the captain of the "rest and digest" aspect of our parasympathetic nervous system. This nervous system allows our muscles to relax, helps us to sleep, helps us digest food, and aids in the body's restoration process. It's the necessary counterpart to the sympathetic nervous system, our "fight, flight, freeze, or fornicate" system. The sympathetic nervous system allows us to deal with high-intensity situations, including life-threatening stressors, in the moment. It helps us orient and focus on specific parts of our environment and decide whether and how to take action—for example, by increasing blood flow to the muscles and helping them contract and increasing our heart rhythm to prepare us to fight, flee, freeze, or take other action.

These two parts of our nervous system (sympathetic and parasympathetic) are always working together. Think of them as the yin and yang of the nervous system—the parasympathetic nervous system fosters greater relaxation and receptivity, and the sympathetic nervous system fosters direction and action. Both aspects of the nervous system are necessary, and their balance of activity is key to our health.

Unfortunately, our world seems to put us in sympathetic overdrive. Our overactive bodies and minds, combined with feelings of anxiety and stress, often cause our sympathetic nervous system to dominate the scene. That leads us to have problems such as increased muscle tension and pain, inability to sleep, and inflammation in our bodies. However, when we can activate our vagus nerve at will, we can help reduce the effects of sympathetic overdrive by bringing our relaxation responses more prominently to the forefront. The vagus nerve helps to keep the sympathetic nervous system in balance so that we don't fall into exhaustion and poor health from overdoing it.

If you ever saw the vagus, you'd wonder how such a seemingly meandering pathway could have the "nerve" to accomplish so many goals within the body! It visits so many friends—how could it possibly get anything done? In fact, this is exactly how the vagus is able to exert its influence. The vagus connects to and networks the brain with the heart, gut, spleen, intestines, liver, and kidneys. In this way, the brain (which many might describe as the CEO of the body) can also "talk to" and influence organs and immune cells via the vagus. The firing of brain cells influences the firing of the vagus nerve. The firing of cells in the vagus nerve in turn directs the organs how to behave—for example, the heart to beat more slowly, the breath to slow down, and even the stomach and intestines to regulate the pace of digestion.

But it's not just a one-way street where the brain influences these organs via the vagus. If the brain has been thought of as the CEO of the body, giving top-down instructions to the organs to act in particular ways, then the vagus is the hard-working managing director, who engages in two-way communications with all the organs and even (gasp) shares advice from the organs upon which the "brainy" CEO might act. Having both sensory and motor fibers, the vagus nerve can both take in information from many of these organs and send signals to direct the brain to behave in particular ways.

For example, the vagus also plays a huge role in helping the immune system and the brain communicate. Key to this communication are little proteins called cytokines.[51] Cytokines can be thought of as neurotransmitters of the immune system. Like neurotransmitters released by neurons, cytokines are proteins secreted by immune cells, including in the lungs, the gastrointestinal (GI) tract, and the heart. Our bodies have a balance of both inflammatory cytokines and anti-inflammatory cytokines. Both are needed for our health, and both work together to create the dance of immune health, including what are called our *innate*, or quick-acting, immunity and our *adaptive*, or longer-term, immunity.[52]

When cytokines are released by immune cells from our organs, they are recognized by the vagus nerve, which has connections with these organs. The vagus nerve then signals the brain to influence the release of neurotransmitters such as acetylcholine, dopamine, and serotonin, influencing our moods and behavior. In this way, the activity of organs and the release of cytokines from immune cells in our guts, heart, and lungs can influence our brain function through the vagus nerve. The vagus is thus the bidirectional communication system through which our organs and our brain are in constant sync with each other, creating a mind-body network.

So exactly how does the vagus nerve integrate the effects of mind-body therapies? We know about the mental (sometimes called *top-down*) components of these practices that influence our attention and emotional state. The vagus relays those brain signal changes to the body and might, for example, signal the body to relax when the fear response is dampened down (as seen by reductions in the activation of the amygdala). But we also have body responses (sometimes called *bottom-up*), such as moving and stretching our muscles and changing our breathing, that affect the firing of the vagus nerve and relay that information to the brain. The stretching and alteration of breathing also affect our brain activity. The vagus, then, is the integrator of mind-body practice—linking our bodies and brain responses so that they are in sync. This two-way connection is reflected in figure 6.1.

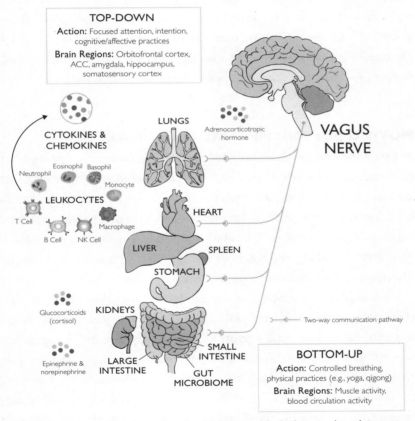

FIGURE 6.1. The vagus nerve plays a role in mind-body therapies through its two-way communication with the brain and body organs. Current research suggests that mind-body therapies have both top-down effects (relating to attention and emotion regulation, reflected by changes in the brain) and bottom-up effects (relating to changes in breathing and movement). Thank you to Dr. Blake Gurfein and Jason Cox for their contributions to this graphic.

WHAT'S QI GOT TO DO WITH IT?

What about the spiritual and energetic levels of healing? What about the role of the biofield in self-healing? The physical mechanisms of healing we explored in the vagus nerve and immune system are fascinating but say little to nothing directly about what the ancient practices considered the central role of prana, qi, or life force in promoting healing. Does this so-called vital life force, or biofield, really have anything to do with healing? If so, can we work with the biofield not only to heal ourselves but also to heal others?

How could we best answer these questions, honoring time-honored practices while still holding to scientific rigor? Could studying the biofield and energy healing give us glimpses into the power of the human healing potential—going even beyond the brain to uncover how subtle energy awareness and spiritual connection can foster healing in others as well as ourselves? Can we work directly with the biofield to help reduce globally rampant suffering from chronic disease, mental disorders, and pain?

MOVING BEYOND MEDITATION RESEARCH

As I went through my clinical psychology training, I witnessed firsthand how grave the need is for evidence-based, nonharmful solutions for problems such as cancer, pain, post-traumatic stress disorder (PTSD), and other ailments. We have already seen that medications such as opioids are not the answer for treating chronic pain. In fact, holistic solutions, including meditation and yoga, are now recommended by the American College of Physicians and others as first-line treatments for such conditions as chronic low back pain.[53]

Although self-care practices are extremely important for us to take charge of our health and maintain a fulfilling life, sometimes life throws us curveballs and we need support. It's not so easy to learn or engage in a new self-care practice when we are in extreme emotional or physical pain. These are times when healing on the emotional, energetic, and spiritual levels becomes every bit as important as on the physical level, and healing connection, or being given a healing "boost," can mean the difference between life or death, as we found in Meera's case in chapter 1. Put simply, when we are in a significantly compromised health state, we have much less energy to engage in self-care practices. We might need a skilled healing practitioner to get us back on the road to healing ourselves.

Although I enjoyed my initial research into mindfulness meditation, it became clear to me that leaders in the field were not going to explore the deeper spiritual aspects of the practice—including the experiences of the biofield. In fact, it seemed we were all dancing around this concept of spirituality without naming the biofield at all. Energetic and spiritual experiences were not discussed in Western-adapted mindfulness practices such as MBSR and mindfulness-based cognitive therapy (I have trained in and used both with patients), although participants were having these experiences. When I asked colleagues why we chose not to discuss energetic or spiritual experiences related to the practices, whether in teaching or in research, I was told it was to secularize them so everyone could access the practices. This is understandable—science has had a history of being oppressed by religion. However, scientists' self-imposed limitations in examining the full picture of these spiritual practices, in my view, has rendered the study and impact of these practices largely incomplete.

If discussing cultural origins and concepts of these practices, including their descriptions of levels of awareness, was of little interest to Western scientists (mostly older Caucasian males), scientifically exploring concepts of the biofield and energy seemed even more threatening. For some, it was too "foreign" (for example, I even had a professor at the University of Arizona describe to me how Ayurveda and the biofield were "primitive medicine"). Other researchers were simply too uncomfortable to explore or discuss anything beyond physical changes to the brain. They were also concerned about their reputations because concepts such as the biofield and energy were still considered "out there."

However, I couldn't help but feel we were missing the point. We weren't, as Western scientists, exploring the deeper spiritual links within these practices and the bridge that linked consciousness with healing. We were content to study brain changes and chalk up the mechanisms of these spiritual practices to cognitive shifts and bodily changes. Some researchers never discussed concepts such as consciousness and how they relate to the healing processes they saw in meditative practice. The field of study of meditation in the early 2000s, to put it bluntly, felt a bit empty.

I decided to apply my training in psychoneuroimmunology and clinical trial research to the study of biofield healing—particularly, examining whether practices such as Healing Touch and laying on of hands could benefit patients struggling with cancer, pain, PTSD, and other issues. Here was a way I could explore the links between spiritual connection and mental/physical/emotional healing—through the biofield. I also thought it was necessary for us as scientists to study these time-honored biofield practices and not dismiss them, particularly for patients suffering significantly. Put simply, from an energetic/spiritual healing point of view, patients who have debilitating amounts of pain, post-traumatic stress, and health challenges such as cancer are often too exhausted to learn and engage in self-care programs such as meditation or exercise. They need connection with loving presence as well as an energy boost to help them get over the hump of their disease process and augment their ability to heal themselves. This is largely what biofield healers do, as we'll learn more about in the coming chapters. I suspected that if we could better understand what these healers were doing and how their work with energy and spiritual presence was fostering healing in patients, we could truly uncover the deeper secrets of healing discussed thousands of years ago and foster significant breakthroughs in how we see, experience, and heal ourselves as spiritual beings having a human experience.

As I sought the answers to these questions through my own research, I came across many more researchers well established in their fields of neuroscience, psychoneuroimmunology, physics, and other disciplines who were interested in answering the same questions. How does consciousness play a role in healing? How does the biofield affect healing, and how does it relate to our abilities to heal others? These scientists were often conducting their experiments in biofield science and healing undercover while doing their mainstream, National Institute of Health (NIH) funded work. But their biofield research was compelling and rigorous. To be frank, the results they were reporting, including clinical trial research, research with cells, and animal model research, were completely mind-blowing in terms of helping us understand that simply working with our energy field can help us recover from disease all the way down to the cellular level. I wondered why the scientific community seemed to turn a blind eye to it.

In the next few chapters, I'll take you on my journey into biofield science and healing, sharing not only the best scientific findings so far but also the stories of these courageous scientists truly dedicated to the discovery of the connection between consciousness and healing. As you sit with what I am sharing with you, I invite you to peruse any of the references to the peer-reviewed, published studies should you question whether the science of biofield healing is real. In my view, the research is just beginning. Despite the incredibly promising findings, significant work must be done in this field. But the data so far are beyond compelling, and if we read and listen closely with our hearts as well as our minds to what the results are telling us, we'll begin to discover just how powerful human beings are as healers not only of ourselves but also of others.

CHAPTER 7

Can We Heal Each Other?
Biofield Therapies and Health

With my initial meditation research as well as my Reiki investigations, I was excited to dedicate my training and research career to exploring mind-body and biofield healing practices. As luck would have it, while I was at the University of Arizona, the National Institutes of Health (NIH) National Center for Complementary and Alternative Medicine (NCCAM; now called the National Center for Complementary and Integrative Health, or NCCIH) released the first (and only) announcement for applications for research centers in biofield science. This announcement was a huge breakthrough for the field. Sadly, though, to the date of this writing, NIH calls for proposals for biofield science and healing research have dwindled to basically nothing, in large part because of perceptions that this work is still too controversial for mainstream science. After a tremendous amount of work by Gary Schwartz and his colleagues and students, we were thrilled to learn his lab was awarded one of the centers. It seemed like the perfect place to conduct my PhD work—except for one thing. None of Schwartz's mentees would be accepted into the clinical psychology program at the University of Arizona.

Schwartz's work was considered controversial by many in academia. Some of his own research interests were in the realm of parapsychology—

particularly what he called *survival of consciousness after death*. While I was at the university, the Clinical Psychology Department asked him to step down from his affiliation with them because they were afraid his controversial research would cause them to lose their accreditation. As a result of his no longer being affiliated with the Clinical Psychology Department, though he was still a faculty member in the Department of Psychology, none of his new students would be admitted into the clinical psychology program.

This was a conundrum for me. I had deeply wanted to be a clinical psychologist as well as a researcher and was planning to apply to transfer into the department's clinical program from the Department of Psychology. I had already been admitted into several other clinical psychology programs, including a prestigious joint doctoral program between San Diego State University (SDSU) and the University of California–San Diego (UCSD)—considered one of the best in the country, with top scientists in psychoneuroimmunology (PNI). At the same time, I had an opportunity to stay and help forward groundbreaking research in biofield healing—but it would cost me my opportunity to work with patients as a clinical psychologist.

TAKING THE LEAP

I ended up following my clinical heart and taking up my deferment to the SDSU/UCSD joint doctoral program in clinical psychology to study there. But before I did, I called up my mentor-to-be at UCSD, Paul Mills, a leading researcher in PNI at the time doing fairly mainstream work in cardiovascular disease and exercise. I knew from talking with him during my interviews at UCSD that he had a deep interest in meditation research and in fact got his PhD in neuroscience from Maharishi International University, where he conducted his doctoral study on the effects of meditation on hormonal influences of heart health. I sensed that although he had taken a fairly mainstream approach in his research up to that point, he had a rich spiritual life. I hoped he might understand my passions and support my growth as a researcher in biofield science.

In this doctoral program, as in many, students were known to simply take up the work of their mentors, examining one of the data sets from a big NIH grant their mentor had received and using that data for their dissertation. This way, students did not have to bear the burden of and take too much time trying to get their own grant and running their own study. They could then graduate more quickly. This pathway was almost expected—in general, graduate students in this program did not rock the boat by trying to conduct their own clinical trial, let alone on something out of the box. Too much innovation, despite what many granting agencies say, is career suicide in academia for a growing researcher.

However, I wanted to do a study of my own in biofield healing—which meant somehow, as a fledgling scientist, getting my own grant to support research in what was still considered a controversial area. To succeed, I needed a mentor who would agree to let me go forward with this work, not try to talk me out of it.

After a few brief exchanges with Paul on the phone, I cut to the chase and blurted out, "I want to do a study in energy healing for my dissertation. If I come there, will you support me to do it?" In his typical cool yet loving way (he was an incredible mentor and is now a dear friend and colleague), he took a breath, exhaled, and said, "Yeah. Yeah, I think we can do that!"

IS BIOFIELD HEALING A PLACEBO? THE RANDOMIZED PLACEBO-CONTROLLED TRIAL JOURNEY

The rest was herstory (well, my story). The long and the short of it was, with Paul's guidance, mentorship, and support, and an excellent research and clinical training program, I applied for and received an NIH grant to do the first (and sadly, still the only) clinical trial on biofield healing at UCSD. I examined via a placebo-controlled, randomized clinical trial (RCT) whether energy healing would decrease fatigue and improve hormonal function in breast cancer survivors—and, if so, whether the effects could be attributed to placebo factors.

It wasn't always easy, and Paul often had to go to bat for me. He once told me of a crucial meeting that took place at UCSD's General Clinical Research Center (GCRC), where the study was to take place. Even though I had gotten an NIH grant and obtained ethics approval for the study, the GCRC review group had to agree to have the study conducted there, or it would not happen.

Paul listened to several in the group scoff about the "hocus pocus" of energy healing and how because it wasn't "real," this proposed study was essentially nonsense. After some time, he evenly replied, "Given that many cancer patients are using these therapies, don't we have an obligation to conduct research on them to see whether or not they work and report back to the patients?" His statement was the deciding factor. We got permission to proceed.

I had designed the study to address what everyone at the time felt was the million-dollar question—is energy/biofield healing real or just a placebo? I had learned, as I shared with you in chapter 5, of the power of placebo. Certainly, placebo elements such as expectations, conditioning, relationship, and ritual all played a role in any healing, and those elements were present in energy/biofield healing. Could energy healing simply be attributed to a magnified placebo effect? I was dying to find out.

CANCER-RELATED FATIGUE: IS BIOFIELD HEALING A SOLUTION?

One thing was for certain—we had to figure out what we could do for fatigued breast cancer survivors, because they were going through substantial, needless suffering with no clear options for relief. Most likely you or someone you are close to has been touched by cancer. If so, you've probably seen firsthand how big an issue fatigue is for cancer patients. Certainly fatigue is significant for those receiving chemotherapy and radiation, after which 80 to 90 percent of patients experience fatigue.[1] What we might not realize is that more than one-third of cancer survivors who are not even going through active treatment anymore still suffer from debilitating fatigue—even up to ten years afterward.[2] This fatigue keeps these survivors from functioning well. They don't have enough energy to do basic things such as cooking, spending time with family, or exercising, even if they were used to exercising before.

Still little is known about how to adequately treat this cancer-related fatigue. In fact, when the word got out about my research, I got random calls from cancer survivors all across the country who simply wanted to thank me for conducting a study to help figure out what they could do to decrease their cancer-related fatigue. "My doc doesn't know what to do for me except give me an antidepressant," one patient related. "But I don't have depression. I'm just really wiped out. I'm really glad you're trying to get to the bottom of this."

Clearly, modern allopathic medicine and science still didn't have all the answers when it came to cancer-related fatigue. We understood there were elevations in inflammatory markers and hormone dysregulation for these patients. But no one seemed able to find a drug that would fix the problem—and that wouldn't cause other risks for these cancer survivors, many of whom were still taking hormone therapy drugs such as Tamoxifen.

But from a biofield healing and holistic medicine point of view, the explanations were fairly simple. These patients were simply exhausted. The physical, psychological, and social consequences of having cancer and going through treatment had depleted their stores of energy. From a healing practitioner's perspective, these fatigued survivors were also likely unwittingly holding on to elements they no longer needed in their biofield—whether residues of chemotherapy treatment, psychological anxiety, or other issues. Their vital energy, prana, or chi was at a low ebb. My thought was that biofield healing would help by replenishing their own vital energy force.

HOW HEALING WORKS: WHAT PRACTITIONERS SAY

How would a biofield healing practitioner help a cancer patient with fatigue? From my own work and discussion with healing practitioners, I knew there were some commonalities among how healers envisioned the process of healing and what they believed they were doing. First, they all said the same thing: *they* were not the healers. (Some, quite frankly, don't like to be called "healers" and would rather be called "healing facilitators" to dispel the myth that they are special beings with special powers that aren't accessible to everyone.) Healing practitioners share that they are simply facilitating a process so that a patient can better help heal him- or herself. Healing practitioners say their job is to help realign the person with their spirit or soul through fostering a clearing of any stuck or stagnant energy in the person's biofield. They believe this stagnation is preventing the person from accessing his or her own vital energy force. (The idea of biofield patterns that can either inform or prevent healing is not unlike the concept of *samskaras*, or mental formations, in Eastern spiritual traditions.)

Healing practitioners also generally engage in consciousness-expanding practices to ready themselves for healing—which could be viewed as similar to a meditative process.

What does that preparation practice generally look like for a healer? Here are some of the common elements nearly all healers I've talked to share about how they prepare themselves before doing healing work.

Grounding and Centering

Generally speaking, before healing practitioners work, they bring their consciousness fully into their bodies and make a connection with the Earth as well as with their spiritual guides. (We discuss several ways you can do this for yourself in part III because these powerful approaches also help bring about self-healing.) Grounding and centering allow the practitioner to open to the Consciousness larger than their conditioned selves (whether they call this Consciousness, *universal life energy*, *Spirit*, *God*, or *nature*) to allow healing to happen through them. Although they might focus on particular techniques, healing practitioners understand that the energy flowing through them for healing is not their own—it is Divine energy. They are simply opening themselves up to this Divine flow of energy to foster healing in the patient.

Connecting and Obtaining Permission

Before even touching patients, healing practitioners make sure they connect with their own Source on a spiritual as well as physical level. What does that mean? Practitioners, of course, verbally ask the patients for permission to work on them and do so only with explicit verbal permission. But they also ask for the patients' soul, spirit, or higher selves to participate in the healing. They might also invite any spiritual guides or ancestors of the patients who wish to be present to aid or witness the healing.

Setting Intention, Attention, and Will to Foster Healing

Before healing practitioners begin their work, they also set clear intentions for the healing. Often, practitioners ask Divinity for the healing to be for the patients' best and highest good or for it to foster the patients' realignment with their higher selves. Practitioners also set their attention on the patients' biofields and often use their hands or eyes to sense the patients' energy flow and potential blockages in their biofields (this process is often called *scanning*). Finally, practitioners might use specific techniques to willfully move energy in and around the body, to clear stuck patterns, and to stimulate energy flow anywhere they sense blockages.

These are common steps healing practitioners across traditions take to get ready for healing their patients. From there, protocols and techniques can vary between healing traditions. But beyond this general preparatory process of grounding, asking for permission, tuning in to patients' biofields, and setting an intention to willfully work with energy to foster healing—was there a particular technique that could be used specifically to address cancer-related fatigue?

I went to my healing teacher, Reverend Rosalyn Bruyere, to find out. Rosalyn is a highly regarded healer, often considered a "grandmother of healing," known for her often miraculous successes with patients, including those with cancer. Her techniques have been integrated into biofield healing schools, including Healing Touch and Therapeutic Touch. I had first met her when she was teaching healing to the medical fellows at Andrew Weil's Center for Integrative Medicine at the University of Arizona. In addition to teaching medical professionals how to heal, Rosalyn has collaborated in healing research since the 1970s. She was a coinvestigator in biofield research with Valerie Hunt at the University of California–Los Angeles (UCLA) and collaborated on research with Elmer Green and other pioneering biofield researchers. I asked Rosalyn if she would collaborate with me on my study. Although she was not thrilled with the placebo-controlled research design, she agreed to advise on the healing approach and ensure that the healers in the study were using the approach appropriately. She suggested we use a general process called *chelation*. She wasn't referring to physical chelation but energetic chelation—in which fully clothed patients would lie quietly on a massage table and be touched lightly by the healing practitioners. The practitioners were not giving them a massage and were not using specific acupressure points. The practitioners were simply laying hands on the patients, starting from the feet, all the way up the body to the head, in a specific pattern.

During the practitioners' laying on of hands on the patients' feet and legs especially, they would focus on "getting into the bone." Rosalyn described this as feeling all the way into the body, down to the bone, to "stimulate bone-marrow chi." Practitioners would focus not only on getting into the bone but also on moving energy through the body by detecting balances and imbalances in the patient's biofield and energetically creating "flow" in their biofield where energy was blocked. This practice helped to release any stuck energy and draw out any residual toxicity.

What? Getting into the bone? How could practitioners place their hands on patients' legs and feel down to the bone, stimulating bone-marrow chi? Having had some of my own experiences with healing and understanding what ancient philosophies and medical systems said about the energetic components of healing, I had some inkling of what she was saying, but my scientific mind continued to cogitate. Were we truly "energetic beings" who responded to this type of biofield healing? How did we know that these healing rituals—including the beliefs and expectations of the healing practitioners themselves—were not simply elaborate ways to elicit excellent placebo responses in the patients? Certainly, many of my scientific colleagues were convinced biofield healing was all placebo and no reality. They weren't basing their opinions on the data but only on their assumptions. How could we know for sure?

I could not let go of the burning million-dollar question about whether biofield healing was simply a placebo. I wanted to find out the truth for myself and thought this would be a start; I was fairly certain I would find something of value for these cancer survivors with this study. Could scheduling in rest twice a week and being touched by a friendly practitioner provide health benefits for these women? Could energy/biofield healing itself offer something even more helpful beyond the positive placebo responses from healing expectations, nurturing therapeutic environments, and relaxation? If so, how would it work? I decided to set up the study to carefully address each placebo element to help determine the answer.

We asked fatigued breast cancer survivors done with their treatment as recently as six months previously to as long as ten years previously (whether chemotherapy, radiation, or surgery), but still suffering high levels of fatigue, to be part of the study. We wanted to see whether biofield healing would reduce their fatigue and whether placebo elements such as expectations, touch, and rest might drive the effects. Most RCTs involve at least two groups, and mine included three. Members of the waitlist control group received no additional treatment but just went on with any therapies they were already getting. They were told that at the end of the study, they would be able to receive healing sessions as a thank-you for their participation (hence the waiting list). Another group received biofield healing (which we called hands-on healing) from trained healing practitioners. These healing practitioners each had at least four years of experience working with patients, many of them cancer patients. They performed the chelation exactly as Rosalyn had instructed, for one hour per session, two times a week, for four weeks, for eight sessions total.

In addition, a placebo-control or "mock-healing" group experienced only the effects of touch, rest, and therapeutic interaction the biofield patients were having with the practitioners. This way, we could see whether the effectiveness of the energy practitioners could be better explained by these placebo elements, which members of the placebo-control group would be having as well—without the energy healing. For the mock practitioners, I selected healthy female scientists matched to the healing practitioners by age and gender (the healing practitioners were all female). These scientists delivering the mock healing had no experience in giving or receiving energy healing, and they did not practice meditation, qigong, or yoga. They didn't really believe in energy healing, but they weren't fervently opposed to the idea. They were true skeptics. I trained them in the hand positions the healers were using so that the sequence of touching and the timing were exactly the same. I also told them not to intend to heal the patients but simply to gently touch them and spend time during the hour thinking about their scientific projects, papers, and tasks they needed to do. To an outside observer, it would look like the mock healers and the healing practioners were implementing the same practices.

WHAT'S THE DIFFERENCE BETWEEN A REAL HEALER AND A MOCK HEALER?

However, many biofield healers took issue with this study design. They explained that the biofield isn't simply something only a healer has access to—everyone has one, and, therefore, a study can never control for the biofield itself. "Energy current flows from a higher potential to a lower potential, or in this case, from a healthy organism to the more unhealthy one," Rosalyn explained.[3] "Therefore, your study is not really controlling for 'energy' versus 'no energy.' It's not like the mock practitioners don't have a biofield. If they are healthy and the cancer survivor is not, and if they are touching the survivors for an hour, current is going to go from the mock practitioner to the fatigued survivor, even if they aren't trained in healing. It's just basic principles of energy flow."

I understood what she was saying and recalled my discussions with the Reiki researchers at the University of Arizona, who felt the same way about placebo-controlled designs for their research, arguing that a placebo group does not control for energy, or the biofield. In addition to this, many scientists have also argued that RCTs do not have the best designs to understand holistic healing, whether it's biofield healing, acupuncture, meditation, or even yoga—and these points are valid.[4] For example, RCTs often don't generalize to the regular population because the inclusion criteria are strict so that many patients are excluded if they have comorbidities, or multiple health conditions. In reality, however, most patients have more than one health condition, so those types of people aren't represented in the RCTs.

Treatments in RCTs aren't often reflective of how patients are treated in the real world. For example, I chose to take just one healing technique and study it, and I made all the practitioners and patients do the sessions in silence to minimize the effects of verbal connection, which could be therapeutic in and of itself. I made sure all the sessions were in the same room in a university clinic. In reality, though, healing sessions are done with practitioners who have freedom to use different techniques during the hour as they see fit, who talk with the patients as they see fit, and who might play music or have a room more conducive to relaxation than a busy university clinic. All of these elements can have therapeutic benefit for patients. However, if we were interested in knowing whether biofield healing was better than a placebo, we had to do a controlled study, keeping other conditions the same (such as the room, the nature of the interaction, and the healing technique) to answer the question.

I surmised that even if the placebo-control group was not controlling for the biofield per se, it was still controlling for experience with healing, intention, and technique. The healing practitioners were working with a different frame of consciousness, level of experience, and technique than that of the skeptical scientists told just to touch and tune out. Per the healing practitioners' explanations, in addition to the chelation technique, which allowed them to feel down to the bone and stimulate bone-marrow chi, they were engaging in a self-generated consciousness-expanding process so that they could help augment the healing process in the patients, and they were willfully directing their attention and intention toward fostering healing in the patients by sensing and working with their biofields. So, essentially, beyond the placebo, we were testing the effects of the biofield healing process—the healing intention and willful engagement with the biofield to foster that outcome, with the advantage of years of training in the technique specifically targeted at cancer-related fatigue.

Because the patients wouldn't know whether they were assigned to the real healing practitioners or the mock healer scientists, we told the patients that if they were assigned to a treatment group (not the control group), they would receive sessions that would either be energy healing or touch alone (the mock healing). We explained that we wouldn't tell them which group they were in until the study concluded. To make sure their expectations for getting better would be similar, we told them that both types of treatments (energy healing and touch alone) had been found in studies to foster relaxation. I also made sure all of the treatment sessions were conducted in silence because I didn't want any possible differences between the groups related to their dialogue or therapeutic interactions.

I couldn't stop there, though. I was relatively obsessed with knowing whether the patients' ongoing perceptions of treatment benefit were shaping their responses to the treatment. So, after each treatment session, whether the patients were in the energy-healing or the touch-alone group, I had them take a questionnaire that asked them specific questions: Did they think they were getting energy healing or touch alone? Did they feel that the treatment was helping them with their immunity and well-being? How friendly were their practitioners? How connected did they feel to their practitioners? They rated all of these on a one-to-five scale. I also asked the energy healing practitioners and mock healers to answer questions after each session, including: What were they focusing on during the silent hour of touching the patients? How connected did they feel with their patients? How much did they feel that what they did helped the patients? I put all of these variables into my data analysis to see if they would explain the results.

A SURPRISING DISCOVERY

Some of my results were somewhat predictable, and some were astounding. First, our "blinding" was successful—it turned out participants couldn't guess which group (energy healing or touch alone) they had been assigned to. (Most thought they were in the biofield healing group regardless of which group they were actually in.) Women in both the energy healing and mock groups said that they experienced strong feelings of connection with their practitioners and felt that their treatments were helping them.

What floored me first was the effectiveness of the treatment. These breast cancer survivors were selected because they had high levels of fatigue that wouldn't go away even after treatment—some of them had been suffering with that fatigue for up to ten years. Yet, when compared with members of the waitlist control group, who went on with their lives and treatments as usual, the levels of fatigue in the women in the healing group dropped to what you would expect for a regular person walking down the street—their fatigue remitted to completely normal levels in a month's time, after only eight one-hour healing sessions.[5] This was not only a statistically significant effect but also a highly significant clinical effect (see figure 7.1).

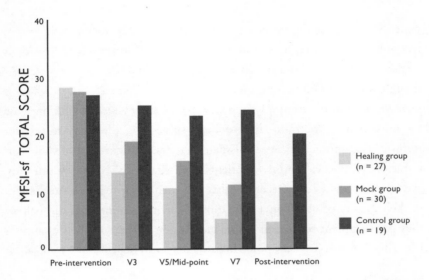

FIGURE 7.1. Changes in fatigue using the Multidimensional Fatigue Symptom Inventory for breast cancer survivors during the four-week study for all three groups. V = visit, with eight one-hour sessions (visits) completed for a four-week period. The healing group (lightest bar) showed a significant and steady decline in fatigue (p < .0005; Cohen's d = 1.04) over the four-week period, compared with the waitlist control group (darkest bar). The mock group (grey bar) also showed a significant decline in fatigue over the four-week period (p = .02, Cohen's d = .68) compared with the waitlist control group. There were also significant differences in general fatigue between the biofield healing and the mock group, with the healing group showing greater decreases in general fatigue compared with the mock group (p = .03, not shown). The full scientific publication can be found in the journal *Cancer*.

What about members of the mock, placebo-control group? Their fatigue dropped significantly too, compared with that of women in the waitlist control group, but not as much as that of the energy healing group members. There was also a statistically significant difference in general fatigue between the energy healing and mock healing groups, with the energy healing group showing greater decreases. Still, compared with members of the waitlist control group, who didn't get any treatment at all, levels of fatigue in the women in the touch-alone group dropped to what you'd expect for a patient with cancer about to go through chemotherapy. This suggested that elements such as positive interactions in a supportive environment, rest, and touch were definitely important—but they weren't telling the whole story.

What about placebo factors such as belief? One of the surprising and important parts of the study was that the patients' belief that they were receiving healing is what improved their quality of life. That is, whether the patients were receiving healing or touch alone, if they believed they were receiving healing, they were more likely to report improvements in their quality of life. Belief didn't predict fatigue or anything else, however. Although we saw an interesting trend for a three-way interaction, in which it seemed those in the healing group who believed they received healing saw the most benefit, we didn't have enough subjects in the study to test for statistical significance. However, I share that data in figure 7.2 to show you how powerful belief can be. If patients didn't believe they received healing, even if they were actually receiving that treatment, they reported no changes in their quality of life. Conversely, those receiving healing who did believe they got treatment seemed to report the greatest changes in their quality of life. This shows us just how powerful the gateway of belief can be for healing.

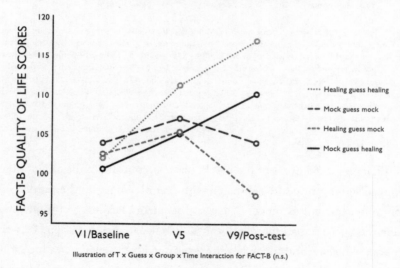

Illustration of T x Guess x Group x Time Interaction for FACT-B (n.s.)

FIGURE 7.2. Data on changes in quality-of-life scores (using the Functional Assessment of Cancer Therapies–Breast QOL Scale) over the four-week study period based on group and treatment belief. Belief in receiving healing significantly predicted quality-of-life scores regardless of whether people were in the healing or mock healing group (p = .04). This figure shows the patterns of belief and quality-of-life changes separated by groups (healing versus mock healing). Although it appeared those who received healing and believed they were getting it increased their scores the most in quality of life, this trend was not statistically significant in our study.

We found the most mind-blowing result, however, when we looked at the physiology. We had measured daily cortisol rhythms in these women.

Although you've probably heard about cortisol as the "stress hormone," it has a number of functions in the body, and, like most hormones, it follows a natural rhythm. Cortisol usually peaks about thirty minutes after you wake up and then steadily declines throughout the day. Generally, when we measure cortisol over time, we see a nice slope, or decrease in cortisol levels, throughout the day.

The rhythm of cortisol is important because it regulates inflammation in the body.[6] Fatigued and depressed breast cancer survivors have been found to have flatter daytime cortisol rhythms.[7] This means their cortisol level does not decrease as much during the day. Sometimes the levels of cortisol go up and down, and sometimes they are just flat, but they don't show that steady decline we want to see showing the body's regulation of the hormone. This lack of cortisol variability, as it is called, appears important clinically—flatter cortisol rhythms have been linked to increased inflammation, and flatter cortisol slopes have been linked to increased risk of death in breast cancer survivors.[8] For our study, cortisol rhythms therefore seemed like an important biomarker to observe. We were interested to know: If healing reduced fatigue, would the cortisol rhythm change as well?

Indeed, we did find a normalization of cortisol rhythms over time—but only for the women in the energy healing group! Those in the touch-alone group and waitlist control groups showed no change at all. When we compared the women in the biofield healing group with those in the mock healing and waitlist control groups, their results were significantly different. I then put other variables into the analysis that could potentially explain the effects, such as body mass index (BMI), prior chemotherapy, and other clinical variables that could affect cortisol rhythms. Even though the study was randomized to try to keep those variables "equal" among groups, could those variables explain the results? Could belief in healing, or connection with the practitioner, predict these results?

No other variables predicted this change in cortisol rhythms. The data basically told me that biofield healing was uniquely affecting these women's fatigue not just psychologically or cognitively but all the way to the hormonal level. But how? I had no idea. By what mechanism was this biofield healing affecting cells? Were there other studies showing similar effects for biofield healing on hormone function or immunity, or was my study a "fluke"?

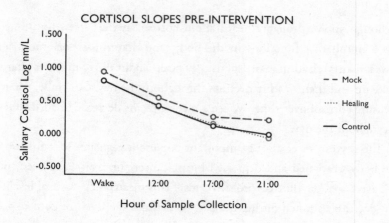

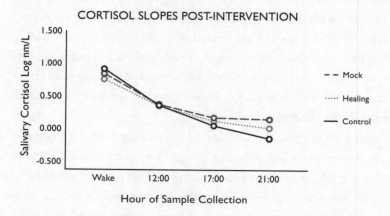

FIGURE 7.3. Slopes of cortisol changes over the day at pre-intervention (before treatments were given) and post-intervention (four weeks later, after eight treatments were given). The energy healing group showed greater changes in cortisol variability (as indexed by more steep slopes) over the four-week period compared with the waitlist control group and the mock healing group (p < .04 in both cases). All details of cortisol capture and data analysis are in the published paper.

FINDING A COMMUNITY OF BIOFIELD SCIENTISTS

I published the study in a well-regarded scientific journal, widely read by on-cologists, called *Cancer*. As I began to present my data at national scientific and health-care conferences, I began to learn more about the work of sever-al senior-level researchers also studying biofield healers, although they didn't necessarily advertise it among their mainstream academic colleagues. I also began to understand how difficult it was for these researchers, many of whom were tenured professors at well-regarded universities and medical centers, to get funding for their research in biofield science or even publish their studies.

For example, around the same time I was conducting my study, Susan Lutgendorf, a professor in the Department of Psychological and Brain Science, Obstetrics and Gynecology, and Urology at the University of Iowa, was conducting a study of a biofield healing approach called Healing Touch for ovarian and cervical cancer patients going through chemotherapy and radiation. She was also conducting a three-group RCT, but it was not placebo controlled with mock healers. Instead, her study compared Healing Touch with another active intervention, relaxation, also thought to have beneficial effects. She randomly assigned patients to receive either Healing Touch, relaxation, or usual care for six weeks while these patients got chemotherapy and radiation. She found that women in the Healing Touch group had significantly reduced depression, whereas the women who received relaxation treatment or usual care did not. In addition, as in my study, she also found a unique effect for Healing Touch on the patient's physiology. She found that only the patients in the Healing Touch group maintained their natural killer-cell function during chemoradiation. Natural killer cells in the immune system not only kill cells with viruses but also help to fight cancer. The natural killer cell function of patients in the relaxation treatment and usual care groups declined as expected during chemoradiation, when immunity is sometimes compromised. But the patients in the Healing Touch group were able to avoid this decline in immunity during chemoradiation by maintaining the function of their natural killer cells.

These results, like mine, seemed mind-blowing. These were *energy therapies, not drugs*—yet they were affecting these cancer patients down to their immune cells. Not only was biofield healing effective for alleviating suffering in cancer patients and survivors by substantially decreasing depression and fatigue but also it uniquely effected changes in their hormones and immune function. The results from these studies suggested this wasn't a result of some nonspecific relaxation or placebo effect because, if so, women in Lutgendorf's relaxation treatment group and women in my mock healing group would have shown changes in their hormone and immune markers. But they didn't. So what was going on? How was biofield healing effecting these changes in the women's bodies?

I began to talk with Lutgendorf and other colleagues about their work—and realized there was even more research going on of which I was not aware because it wasn't being talked about and was essentially being pushed to the side or ignored even when presented at conferences. Despite her ground-breaking findings and the fact that as an established professor well funded by the National Institutes of Health (NIH), National Cancer Institute (NCI), and other agencies for her psychoneuroimmunology research, Lutgendorf was having trouble finding a medical journal that would publish her RCT with Healing Touch for cancer patients. Some journal editors said they just plain didn't believe it. Others said they didn't think it was "rigorous" enough because it wasn't placebo controlled. Lutgendorf finally published her study in a prestigious psychoneuroimmunology journal, although she had hoped to publish it in a broader-based journal so that medical doctors might be more likely to see it.[9]

Yet these data seemed so important. The findings were profound in terms of uncovering human ability to heal others as well as ourselves—down to our cells—as well as showing effects of these low-risk, supportive-care biofield therapies to alleviate needless suffering for patients who had few options. I wondered—how many studies of biofield therapies are there, and what have the results told us so far?

IS BIOFIELD HEALING EFFECTIVE FOR TREATING ILLNESS?

Having conducted my own study and learned about Lutgendorf's, my curiosity was further piqued. How robust are these findings? What do we know about biofield therapies as a whole, in terms of their ability to alleviate suffering for patients with various illnesses? Can healing practitioners foster significant, meaningful changes in patients' suffering simply by working with their biofields? Could healing therapists work successfully alongside other health-care professionals, including nurses and doctors, in clinics and hospitals, to alleviate symptoms in patients with cancer, pain, and other ailments?

I decided to conduct a systematic review, compiling the data across many studies, to determine whether there were consistent, reliable effects of these biofield therapies for patients hospitalized or receiving medical care for Alzheimer's disease, anxiety, cancer, pain, and other ailments. At the time, I compiled and analyzed all the results from sixty-six clinical studies of biofield therapies (including Healing Touch, Johrei, laying on of hands, Reiki, spiritual healing, Therapeutic Touch, and others) that met my rigorous criteria to be included in the study.[10] I used a standardized process to rate each study on quality and evaluated the data based on tried-and-true best-evidence synthesis methods, which draw conclusions about results according to the rigor of each study's research design. Here's what I discovered from that systematic review:

Biofield therapies show strong evidence of reducing pain intensity in patients—beyond a placebo effect. We found thirteen clinical studies of biofield therapies with 979 patients with pain (including patients with arthritis, carpal tunnel, chronic pain, fibromyalgia, neuropathic pain, and osteoarthritis) that examined pain reduction as the main outcome. Nine were RCTs, and seven were placebo-controlled designs. The data showed consistent significant effects of biofield healing therapies on reducing the patients' rating of their pain, with five of the seven placebo-controlled designs showing consistent effects of healing. Our findings are consistent with what others have found—for example, a 2008 *Cochrane* review examined twenty-four RCTs focusing on the effects of Healing Touch, Reiki, and Therapeutic Touch on pain. These other studies reported that these therapies have a significant, modest effect for pain relief (similar to what mindfulness studies report on pain relief), with no statistically significant effects of placebo treatments and no adverse events.[11] Most recently, a meta-analysis of four RCTs was conducted specifically using Reiki for pain relief and reported positive effects.[12]

Biofield therapies show moderate evidence of reducing pain in cancer and hospitalized patients, with more studies needed. What about reducing pain in patients who might be experiencing pain but are not chronic pain patients—such as those who have cancer and those in the hospital? During the time of my review, only four studies examined cancer pain, and only three looked at postoperative pain in hospitalized patients. Based on this limited data, we found moderate evidence for biofield therapies reducing pain in cancer and hospitalized patients. The promise of biofield therapies for cancer pain, but relative lack of sufficient studies, has since been noted by other researchers.[13]

Biofield therapies show promise for improving mental health, but the data are insufficient. In our review, we found a moderate level of evidence that biofield therapies reduced anxiety in hospitalized patients. We also found moderate evidence that biofield therapies reduced agitation symptoms in patients with dementia. However, not many studies had examined the effects of biofield therapies for decreasing anxiety for other patients, such as those with cardiovascular disease and chronic pain. And the few studies published with those patients showed mixed findings. A recent *Cochrane* review on Reiki for anxiety and depression, for example, discovered only three RCTs that met the criteria and found insufficient data to warrant conclusions.[14]

Biofield therapies affect our biology. I already mentioned the findings of my RCT and Lutgendorf's RCT, which showed effects of biofield therapies on hormone function and immune function, independent of placebo or relaxation controls, in cancer survivors and patients. Beyond those studies, other controlled studies have shown that biofield therapy treatments can positively affect blood pressure, brain activation, cortisol rhythm, heart rate, heart rate variability, and salivary IgA levels.[15, 16]

IS TOUCH THE DRIVER OF BIOFIELD HEALING EFFECTS?

Biofield healing practitioners might physically touch the patient, or they might not. In the study I conducted, we used laying on of hands with the Bruyere chelation method, so healing practitioners were touching the patients. However, in many Healing Touch and Therapeutic Touch protocols, as well as in other practices such as Johrei, pranic healing, and external qigong, the practitioners are not touching patients but working with their biofields a few inches off their bodies. My systematic review and other systematic reviews often included all types of healing approaches—regardless of whether patients were being touched. How do we know, then, whether the effects of biofield healing are a result of touch itself? Could the positive results come from being touched?

My colleague Richard Hammerschlag was deeply interested in this question. He decided to conduct a different type of systematic review that looked only at studies in which the healing practitioners were doing the healing without touching (but still in the room with the patients). He found eighteen high-quality RCTs that met his stringent criteria for inclusion in his review. He found that twelve of those eighteen studies showed positive effects in at least one primary outcome—suggesting that positive effects of biofield therapies on clinical outcomes do not simply result from touch.[17] Our nonprofit, the Consciousness and Healing Initiative (CHI), has shared his findings in an interactive infographic that lets you see the data visualization explaining the systematic review process and sort the data yourself by treatment type, gender, age of participant, treatment duration, study design, and more. You can also click on each bubble to gain access to every study—check it out at chi.is/infographic.

WHAT ABOUT ENERGY PSYCHOLOGY, OR "TAPPING," STUDIES?

My review, Hammerschlag's review, and the other reviews I mentioned above included many biofield therapies such as Healing Touch, laying on of hands, Reiki, and others. But at that time, we didn't include other biofield-based therapies such as energy psychology (EP), or "tapping," interventions. Energy psychology treatments include emotional freedom technique (EFT), Tapas acupressure technique (TAT), and thought field therapy (TFT), among others. The practice of energy psychology is different from therapies such as Healing Touch, Reiki, and others. EP techniques are often used within psychotherapy. Instead of sensing and working with the patients' biofields directly, therapists (generally mental health professionals) teach patients how to tap on specific areas of their bodies thought to be points on energy meridians, or pathways of energy, similar to those in acupuncture. Patients learn how to tap their fingers on specific points on these meridians when recalling a troubling event, and therapists guide them through the recalled event. This generally occurs in therapy in which patients are working on particular issues such as unresolved anxiety, phobia, and trauma.

The theory behind EP (not unlike that of many biofield therapies) is that during an anxiety-provoking or traumatic event, people's biofield patterns and their physiology "freeze" in a particular way. Tapping on the meridian points is a conscious way of trying to free any energy frozen during an anxiety-provoking or traumatic incident and thus promotes flow and relaxation into a different physiological state. The Association for Comprehensive Energy Psychology puts it like this: "Within an EP framework, emotional and physical issues are reflected in bio-energetic patterns within and around the mind-body-energy system. Since the mind and body are thought to be interwoven and interactive, this mind-body-energy system involves complex communication involving neurobiological processes, innate electrophysiology, psychoneuroimmunology (PNI), consciousness, and cognitive-behavioral-emotional patterns."[18]

This is all scientific sounding, but is there really any evidence to suggest that tapping on your face and different parts of your body, supposedly shifting your biofield as a result, actually has any effect?

As it turns out, yes—there is evidence that it works. To date, fifty RCTs have been conducted of EP studies alone, along with more than fifty other clinical studies. So far, the synthesis of data over these studies in the form of systematic reviews and meta-analyses focus on EFT in particular. Here is what those systematic reviews and meta-analyses are saying:

EFT is helpful for anxiety and depression. A recent meta-analysis in the *Journal of Nervous and Mental Disorders* examined fourteen studies with 658 participants to determine whether EFT was helpful for anxiety. The authors used the criteria developed by the American Psychological Association's Division 12 Task Force on Empirically Validated Treatments and found studies with patients with phobias, post-traumatic stress disorder (PTSD), and anxiety. The meta-analysis suggested that EFT was substantially and significantly more effective in reducing anxiety compared with control treatments, although the researchers noted that more studies should be conducted comparing EFT to standard-of-care approaches for anxiety such as cognitive-behavioral therapy.[19] Similarly, a different meta-analysis published in the journal *Explore* examined twenty clinical studies (including twelve RCTs) of 859 patients. The authors determined that EFT was significantly effective in substantially reducing depression compared with usual care, but that EFT was no different than eye-movement desensitization reprocessing (EMDR) in relieving depression.[20]

EFT reduces PTSD symptoms. A separate meta-analysis, also published in *Explore*, analyzed seven RCTs examining the effectiveness of EFT specifically for PTSD symptoms and found a substantial and significant reduction in PTSD after four to ten treatment sessions, compared with usual care. Of these RCTs, only two compared EFT to other active treatments, and the data from these two studies suggested no difference between EFT and those treatments for reducing PTSD.[21] Some studies that have found substantial results of EFT for reducing PTSD suggested the results remain over time. A recent RCT, for example, published in the *American Journal of Health Promotion*, showed a more than twenty-five-point decrease in PTSD symptoms for those who received EFT. The significant decreases in PTSD symptoms still remained six months after treatment.[22] This study also reported changes in gene expression for those receiving EFT for PTSD compared with those getting the usual care.

CAN WE HEAL EACH OTHER FROM A DISTANCE?

So far, we've mostly been talking about therapies in which the biofield healing practitioners and the patients are in the same room—whether the practitioners are touching the patients or not. But many practitioners feel that being in the same room has nothing to do with the healing, and they can tune in to and work with patients' biofields even across the world to foster healing. The miraculous healing of Meera, for example, was facilitated by a healer thousands of miles away.

Could this be real, or is this again more of a placebo response in which healing occurs as a result of expectations of receiving healing? Is there evidence across the board to suggest that we can affect people, down to their physiology, from a distance? How robust are the findings?

There are two ways to answer this question. One is to determine, generally, whether a human being can affect people's physiology from a distance, without talking to them or even letting them know that they are tuning in to their biofield (hence not inducing expectations). My friend and colleague Dean Radin, chief scientist at the Institute of Noetic Sciences, describes this type of research as distant mental interaction with a living system (DMILS).[23] DMILS studies allow us to examine, under carefully controlled conditions and robust experimental designs, whether affecting people's physiology from a distance is even possible. The second answer to the question is to examine scientifically through RCTs whether distant healing of patients actually results in beneficial changes for them.

Together, these two fields of research suggest that receiving benefits from distant healing is definitely possible, but it's unclear how strong and how reliable the effects are across the board for different patients, outcomes, and healing traditions. Let's examine DMILS studies—specifically, the effects of distant intention (sometimes called *remote intention*) on people's physiology, first.

Distant intention studies generally involve one sender (S) and one receiver (R) who are not in the same physical location. R is hooked up to a monitor to measure his or her physiology—to give you an idea, physiological outcomes studied in DMILS experiments have included measures such as blood volume pulse, heart rate, skin conductance, and stomach function via the electrogastrogram (EGG). These studies have also looked at brain activity via measures including electroencephalography (EEG), functional magnetic resonance imaging (fMRI), and functional near-infrared spectroscopy (fNIRS).

The experiments are conducted under carefully controlled conditions that typically look like this: The receiver R is simply asked to maintain a state of relaxation and openness for twenty minutes during which some aspect of R's physiology is being recorded. During that time, there are several time blocks, or "epochs," of recording taking place within the twenty minutes—basically the data are time-stamped every thirty seconds. In one thirty-second block, the sender S, who is not in the same physical location as the receiver R and cannot be seen or heard by R, directs attention toward R for thirty seconds with the intention of shifting R's biology. In another block, S simply relaxes for thirty seconds and does not try to tune in to R in the least. The order of blocks in which S sends intention or relaxes is randomized and counterbalanced so that it's not predictable to anyone when S is sending intention to R or when S is relaxing. Each thirty-second epoch, or block, is simply recorded by the computer system. After the recordings are finished for all senders and receivers, the data are sent to a statistician who also doesn't know which blocks involve S sending intention versus S relaxing. The data are then analyzed and later "unblinded" so the investigator can see which blocks (sending versus relaxing) might have shown effects on R's physiology.

These studies have been conducted at several universities around the world, including Lund University in Sweden; Stanford University in California; Cornell University in New York; University of California–Davis; University Hospital in Freiburg, Germany; and more. The most recent, carefully conducted meta-analysis of thirty-six studies of this type, published in the *British Journal of Psychology*, found that first of all, these studies were of strong quality, methodologically speaking. The meta-analysis also found that across the studies, there were statistically significant results supporting the effectiveness of remote intention in changing physiology.[24] However, higher-quality studies showed weaker effects—and still little is known about whether certain body measures might be more likely to change with remote intention than others. Overall, the data at this point are robust enough to conclude that it is possible for human beings to affect another person's physiology from a distance. However, we need more high-quality studies in the area of remote intention to determine just how strong the effects might be and which bodily systems might be most affected by remote intention.

What about studies in which people are intending healing and sending energy to other people from a distance as opposed to affecting some physiological parameter in blocks of thirty seconds? Most healers don't work that way, and many healers have complained that the idea of having on/off periods of thirty seconds (i.e., sending healing for thirty seconds, then stopping, then starting again, etc.) in a research study on healing is just unrealistic and not aligned with the healing practice. If we observe healers in a more natural situation, in which they send healing intention and energy to another person, but from a distance as opposed to being in the same room, do we see effects?

As it turns out, dozens of studies have examined distant healing, and several scientists have synthesized the results at this point. One meta-analysis, published in *Explore*, analyzed the data from forty-nine studies in which researchers looked at distant healing on biological outcomes in nonhuman recipients (including outcomes in bacteria, cancer cells in animals, cells in dishes, plant growth, and yeast). The meta-analysis reported that overall, these studies show significant effects of distant healing on these animal, cell, and plant outcomes.[25]

Conclusions about distant healing in humans have been more ambiguous. One of the first systematic reviews published on distant healing in humans was in 2000 by John Astin and colleagues, in *Annals of Internal Medicine*. This review synthesized data from twenty-three RCTs of 2,774 patients and included studies in intercessory prayer (praying for someone's healing), as well as biofield-based distant healing (such as Reiki and Therapeutic Touch). They found that thirteen of the studies showed statistically significant treatment effects, nine showed no effects, and one showed a negative effect.[26] A few years later, Edward Ernst, one of the original coauthors and a known skeptic of biofield healing, conducted further analyses and challenged this systematic review. Based on his analysis, he claimed that most of the higher-quality studies did not show "specific therapeutic effects," and therefore distant healing is no better than a placebo.[27]

What about prayer? Astin and Ernst's analyses had put prayer and distant healing methods into the same category. However from a scientific and biofield practice point of view, it's unclear whether these can be lumped together. Often praying for someone else's healing does not necessarily mean that the intercessor is tuning in to someone's energy from a distance, scanning for balances and imbalances in the person's biofield, and sending intention to shift his or her energy in a particular way. The process of prayer can be very different from this. Often prayers are simply offered to God or the Divine for the healing of another person, without any intentional process to energetically scan or send energy to the person directly. People who pray for another, although this could certainly be considered a form of healing, might not be trained or even care about the biofield. Do we know anything about the differences between these types of remote healing approaches?

Wayne Jonas, executive director of Samueli Health Programs, and his colleague Cindy Crawford, senior research associate at the Henry Jackson Foundation, have been exploring the effects of biofield healing for decades. In their 2001 meta-analysis, they reviewed thirteen studies of intercessory prayer and nineteen studies of energy healing. They found that both sets of studies had fair methodological quality and that both showed meaningful effects, although the effects were larger for energy healing overall compared with those of prayer.[28]

Another recent meta-analysis by Chris Roe and colleagues at the University of Northampton in the United Kingdom compared intercessory prayer with other distant healing approaches including Johrei, Reiki, and Therapeutic Touch. Roe and colleagues reported that of the twenty-seven studies that met rigorous methodological quality, there were small but significant effects overall on participant well-being compared with those on control subjects who did not receive healing. In line with findings reported by Jonas and colleagues, subanalyses indicated that prayer had smaller effects than did distant healing approaches such as Johrei, Reiki, and Therapeutic Touch.

Other reviews that have compiled the data for intercessory prayer alone suggest that as a whole, as studied, it has not shown significant outcomes for the patients studied. A 2009 *Cochrane* systematic review looked at ten RCTs of intercessory prayer over 7,646 patients with serious illnesses. Most studies had people of Judeo-Christian faith as intercessors, although some studies reported having people of different faiths and traditions offer prayers for patients. The outcomes suggested that intercessory prayer, as studied, had no significant effects on outcomes, including clinical status, death, or readmission to the hospital.[29] Similar results were reported in another independent meta-analysis of prayer in 2006.[30]

Does this mean that praying for another person does not work at all? I do not believe we have the data to answer this question because the research is limited with respect to how we understand and measure healing. It is interesting to me that the prayer studies, meant to examine the effects of spirituality and spiritual experiences in fostering a healing response, are designed with outcomes that prioritize physical "cures" as healing—with no mention of spiritual or even mental and emotional effects. The outcomes assessed in these prayer studies are more about praying for extremely ill patients to prevent their death, further disease, or readmission to a hospital— as if this is all healing is about.

Yet when we ask healing practitioners, including those of Christian and other religious faiths, how healing works, we hear that it is about being made whole and being realigned with a larger Consciousness. It is not necessarily only about getting rid of a disease or preventing readmission to a hospital, which is really all we've looked at in these RCTs. In these studies, the people praying for patients are often asked to pray for people they don't know. Because the focus has been on RCTs to try to "tease out belief," the patients might be told people are praying for them when they really aren't, or they might be told people aren't praying for them when they really are. Are these the appropriate scientific designs to study the sacred?

Healers tell us that the process of healing is about soul or spiritual realignment. The studies reviewed in these meta-analyses didn't look at outcomes that relate to spiritual health as well as emotional, interpersonal, mental, and physical health. To get a fuller picture of healing, whether by prayer, whether by distant healing of biofields, or whether by healing-by-touch practitioners in the same room, we need to look beyond whether prayer keeps someone from death when they are critically ill or whether it changes their medical diagnosis, as if those were the only outcomes that matter. We need to look at the whole person, including emotional health, interpersonal harmony, and spiritual health.

EXTRAORDINARY EXPERIENCES DURING HEALING: LINDA'S STORY

What do patients say about their spiritual experiences while receiving healing? Although some scholars have actually interviewed patients about their healing experiences, many patient stories are never heard because the data collection isn't set up to capture those experiences. Take Linda, for example, a fatigued breast cancer patient in my study. I ended up hearing about Linda's extraordinary healing experience in a CNN episode, after CNN came to the University of California–San Diego (UCSD) to interview us about our study.

Linda was part of the mock healing, or placebo-control, group in our study. After she had finished participating in the study and we collected all the official data outcomes, in gratitude for her being part of the study, we offered her, as well as all other participants in the mock healing group and waitlist control group, three healing sessions with Janet, one of our trained biofield healing practitioners, at no cost. We thought all the women in the study should get the opportunity to experience the actual hands-on healing if they wanted to. Linda elected to receive the healing sessions after her part in the study was completed. The CNN interviewers were excited to interview Linda because they were interested in whether Linda saw differences between the mock healing and the biofield healing she received.

In her interview with CNN, Linda noted that she had felt relaxed during the mock healing sessions but that something extraordinary had happened during the healing with Janet: "I could feel energy being moved in my body. I could feel resistance in a portion of my body, and afterward I asked the practitioner about what was going on. She told me that she was getting a message from my mother—but the practitioner knew nothing about me."

Janet was getting a message from Linda's deceased mother, whom she had never met or known about. The message from Linda's mother, meant for Janet to pass along to Linda, was that for a long time Linda's mother had felt that her work with Linda was not complete.

"My mother recently died. She was eighty-four years old. She was the one who took care of me during my breast cancer," Linda shared. "She really did . . ." Linda tearfully took a few moments before she spoke next about the tremendous sense of resolution that came through the healing. "Her work with me was finished because she saw me through my reconstruction . . . and she was now able to see that I was doing well. That was very powerful for her . . . the practitioner . . . to be that aware."

Stories like this are not uncommon. Healers often report that deceased loved ones or ancestors of patients are present during a session to help guide the healing or simply to support patients. Often, healers report, these loved ones have a message they wish for the healer to pass along to the patient. But sometimes the patients get those messages directly or have extraordinary spiritual experiences.

Some scholars have interviewed patients about their experiences with healing, using qualitative interviews and coding their responses into data they analyze. Those studies of different types of biofield healing approaches have reported that patients receiving healing often have unusual sensory experiences (including feeling energy in the body and seeing light), feeling a strong sense of connection with Spirit or God, and feeling or seeing spiritual beings during the healing.[31]

Reports of patients' experiences like these help us to remember the real value of biofield healing approaches for just about anyone. These therapies are bringing us closer to the depths of Consciousness. From there, many outcomes are possible, which might or might not include physical healing.

As a scientist in this field, I was taught to think that the most valuable action I could take was to "prove" that healing exists by showing its effectiveness in changing biomarkers in the body or "prove" that healing exists beyond placebo effects. Because most scientists' fascination and focus is on the physical, healing is somehow seen as more "real" if it results in changes in brainwaves or immune cells as opposed to changes in emotional, mental, or spiritual states. But we might forget that our emotional, interpersonal, mental, physical, and spiritual well-being are connected—they are all aspects of us as whole human beings. As we explored earlier, findings in psychoneuroimmunology show us just how powerful our emotional, interpersonal, and mental health are for our bodies. So looking at all aspects of the whole person is important. Healing isn't just about getting rid of a disease. It's about providing peace and returning the person to a state of wholeness. That might be the most powerful aspect we can really examine about the promise of these healing approaches, especially in today's times.

So how many total biofield healing studies with patients are there?

Since the time of my comprehensive review in 2009, more than 170 clinical trials of biofield therapies have been published, many of them RCTs. I've already explored in detail two of the RCTs (my study on fatigued breast cancer survivors and Lutgendorf's study on ovarian and cervical cancer patients going through chemoradiation). Many of the newer studies have been published outside of the United States, including in countries such as Brazil, France, and Spain. In general, although there are not thousands of clinical studies on biofield therapies, there are hundreds. When we recently searched for peer-reviewed, published, scientific, clinical studies of biofield therapies alone, we found a total of more than 400 clinical studies, including more than 125 RCTs, on biofield therapies (including energy psychology).

If you're new to this area of biofield science and healing, you might be pondering what I've been saying in this chapter. You might still feel doubtful about whether there is a "there there" in energy healing—after all, I only shared results from a few RCTs with you, and even though I've summarized results that suggest healing another person's biofield seems to work beyond what we call a placebo effect; that it actually has clinically significant effects; and that it even affects functions such as heart rate, hormone rhythm, and immune cells and even fosters spiritual experiences in people, this might all still seem unbelievable. Can we really heal another person without drugs, needles, talk therapy, or even stretching? If so, how does it really work? After all, I haven't said anything about how we might measure the biofield, so how do we know the biofield really has anything to do with it? Even if you are more familiar with this work, you might wonder—what is it about connecting with the energetic and the spiritual in this way that can affect us all the way down to our cells? How powerful is this energy with which we can all send healing?

Although, as I've said above, healing is not just about altering the physical—I appreciate that believing healing is possible is just more resonant when we actually see those changes on the physical level. It also helps us understand how much there still is to learn about how consciousness, through the biofield, is shifting biology. I certainly wondered, and still do, about how the biofield bridges the physical and the spiritual. So when I found out about the carefully controlled studies my scientific colleagues were doing—not with humans but with cells and with animals—and seeing really incredible shifts in results such as cell growth, improved cell function, and decreased tumor size—all with biofield healers—I had to learn more. Let's explore these discoveries in chapter 8.

CHAPTER 8

Healing Down to Our Cells

I can still remember when I stumbled into a presentation by Gloria Gronowicz, a professor of surgery and orthopedic surgery at the University of Connecticut, at the International Research Congress on Integrative Medicine and Health in 2010. While Harvard researcher Ted Kaptchuk gave a captivating ninety-minute morning keynote to hundreds of people on the history of placebos, in a small room with a handful of people present, Gronowicz gave a ten-minute presentation on her groundbreaking, placebo-controlled study showing that Therapeutic Touch (TT), as compared with mock TT, influenced the growth of bone, tendon, and connective tissue cells.

Gronowicz, known and funded by the National Institutes for Health (NIH) for her more mainstream work on the process of bone formation, was also interested in exploring how biofield healing, specifically TT, might affect the growth of cells that help make connective tissue (fibroblasts and tenocytes) and cells that help make bone (osteoblasts).[1]

Gronowicz recruited three TT practitioners for the study. All were registered nurses (as are many TT practitioners) who had five or more years of experience using TT with patients. In designing her study, Gronowicz was interested in knowing whether any positive results she might find could be a result of a person's general physical presence or movement of hands around a cell dish. To control for this possibility, she also recruited four scientists with no experience in TT who would mimic the hand positions of the TT practitioners but without intent to heal. While providing this sham treatment, the scientists were instructed to mentally count backward by fours from the number 1,000 to keep their minds occupied.

TT practitioners treated cells from a distance of fifteen inches for ten minutes twice a week for two weeks; the scientists performed the sham control procedure at a similar distance and for the same amount of time. After all treatments were completed, technicians "blinded" to the treatment groups (i.e., they didn't know if the cells were treated by TT practitioners or mock healers) analyzed the cell growth counts.

The results revealed that the TT-treated cells (bone, tendon, and connective tissue) significantly increased in number when compared with the cells in the sham control procedure.[2]

Gronowicz then wondered whether TT was specific in its effects on cell growth. Would it increase the number of all types of cells, whether cancerous or normal, or was the biofield effect "intelligent," leaning in the direction of promoting healing? She set up a similar procedure, this time specifically testing how TT influenced human osteoblasts, cells that promote the formation and mineralization of bone. In the same study, she also examined how TT influenced bone cancer (osteosarcoma) cells.

In this study, Gronowicz found something astounding. As in her previous study, TT increased the DNA synthesis, cell differentiation, and mineralization in regular bone cells, but it had the opposite effect on bone cancer cells. In these cells, TT significantly decreased cell differentiation and mineralization.

I remember just being amazed when I saw these results. I went up to Gronowicz, whom I did not know at the time, and introduced myself. "These are amazing findings!" I exclaimed. "I hope you will publish them and extend this work further."

Gronowicz thanked me for my interest and my own research, and she also shared her story about how she was able to conduct this research. These studies, along with Susan Lutgendorf's Healing Touch randomized controlled trials (RCTs) with cancer patients, were part of the same type of NIH National Center for Complementary and Alternative Medicine (NCCAM) grant for biofield science that Gary Schwartz and his colleagues at the University of Arizona had received. But even after these grants allowed for the publication of this promising research, NCCAM did not follow through with an additional grant to extend the findings. There was notable pressure on NCCAM from skeptics who insisted that TT was nonexistent energy healing and therefore "quackademic medicine." Perhaps as a result of the bad press, NCCAM downplayed its involvement in this area of research and decided not to prioritize further funding in biofield science. This basically created a financial roadblock, preventing credible, interested scientists from conducting rigorous research in biofield healing.

Gronowicz also shared with me that she was having trouble publishing her study in mainstream medical journals. When submitting her manuscripts for publication, she was shocked at the pushback because the reticence to publish her findings had little to do with the soundness of her design or the methodology in carrying out the research and analyzing the data. Gronowicz actually wrote to the editor of one of the journals in which she often published her more mainstream work, noting, "If I was reporting these results with a drug, you would have no trouble publishing this." Because of her persistence, much like Lutgendorf, eventually she was able to get some of her TT data published in a mainstream journal, the *Journal of Orthopedic Research*.[3] Her other studies were published in integrative medicine journals—good, credible journals, but they don't necessarily reach people in mainstream medicine.

BIOFIELD THERAPIES AFFECT CANCER BIOLOGY: UNCOVERING IMMUNE PATHWAYS IN MOUSE MODELS

Gronowicz's studies weren't the only ones showing differential effects of biofield therapies on cancer cells as compared with normal cells. Harvard University researchers who had collaborated with qigong grand master and physician Yan Xin revealed similar findings when Yan Xin emitted qigong energy for healing purposes. In one study, for example, the Harvard researchers found that just five minutes of emitted qigong on pancreatic cancer cells moved the cells to dismantle (specifically, it induced apoptosis, or cell death, and increased the sub-G1 cell population, DNA fragmentation, and cleavage of caspases 3, 8, and 9 and poly[ADP-ribose] polymerase). In longer-term qigong emission studies, the energy also caused the pancreatic cancer cells to lyse (die). Interestingly, just as in Gronowicz's study with cancerous and noncancerous cells, researchers found no cell destruction or enzymatic changes in similarly treated normal cells.[4]

For those of you who want more cellular details, here are some additional findings: The researchers found that qigong energy emission inhibited the activity of particular protein kinases (basal Akt and ERK1/2). Protein kinases are enzymes that regulate the biological activity of proteins by phosphorylating them with ATP to create a conformational change in the protein. That conformational change is what makes a protein go from being inactive to active. Think of a protein kinase as regulating part of the chain of protein changes that drive cell behavior, including cell growth and survival. In cancer cells, increased activity of the kinases Akt and ERK1/2 is related to increased pancreatic cancer growth, survival, and resistance to chemotherapy.[5] Inhibiting these kinases thus seems promising for helping treat pancreatic cancer—in fact, some researchers are also investigating how drugs might inhibit these kinases to treat cancer.[6]

However, no drug was needed to inhibit this protein kinase pathway—in this case qigong energy significantly and substantially reduced the activity of these protein kinases in pancreatic cancer cells, and there was increased apoptosis of the cancer cells. But in qigong emission to noncancerous, normal fibroblasts (connective tissue cells), the activity in these enzymes *increased* as opposed to decreasing. This suggests that the qigong biofield therapy specifically and differentially affected cell death in cancerous versus noncancerous cells. Again, the emitted qigong energy seemed to have a kind of "intelligence." This research group went on to demonstrate similar effects on breast cancer, colorectal cancer, and prostate cancer cells.[7]

One might wonder: If qigong therapy seemed to have specific effects in lysing cancerous cells in a dish, what could biofield therapies do to the cellular structure of cancer tumors in a living being? Could they prevent tumor growth and tumor spread, and if so, how? To further examine the potential effects of biofield therapies on cancerous cells, Gronowicz conducted her next study on mice. In this study, she had control mice that received a saline injection and mice injected with 66c14 breast cancer cells. She then treated a subset of the cancerous mice with real TT and another subset with sham TT, as in her other studies.

Gronowicz's results seemed incredible but perhaps not surprising given the findings of her previous studies and the Harvard qigong emission studies. The mice treated with real TT, but not the mice treated with mock TT, showed reductions in cancer metastasis (cancer tumor migration). Cancer spread was inhibited with TT, but how?

Gronowicz looked more deeply at the immune systems of these mice. It seemed the real biofield therapy, but not the sham therapy, was profoundly affecting their cancer. She noticed that when she injected mice with cancer, levels of eleven cytokines (immune transmitters often involved in inflammation and sometimes in cancer cell growth and migration) increased substantially and significantly when compared with cytokine levels in the control mice not injected with cancer. Then the mice with cancer were treated with either TT or sham TT. Those receiving TT over two weeks showed reductions in four of these inflammatory cytokines, specifically interleukins 1a and 1b (IL-1a and IL-1b), macrophage inflammatory protein-2-alpha (MIP-2), and monokine-induced gamma interferon (MIG)—down to levels found in the control mice. This result was also significantly different in the mice treated with mock TT, which showed no such reductions in these cytokines.

Gronowicz also found that mice treated with TT showed changes in certain immune cell subsets related to breast cancer in one of the first preclinical studies.[8] Specifically, TT decreased certain white blood cells called *lymphocytes* related to tumor migration (CD44hiCD25 and CD44hiCD25-, in the spleen, and CD44loCD25+, in the lymph node) compared with those in both the mice treated with sham TT and the control mice. The results suggested that TT reduced cancer metastasis by reducing the number of cells and immune transmitters involved in tumor migration.

Gronowicz then attempted to repeat these findings. What would happen if she gave mice TT before they were even injected with cancer cells?

Would receiving TT before getting cancer have a preventative effect? She repeated her study, but this time, in addition to treating the mice after they had been injected with cancer, the TT practitioners also pretreated the mice with TT before they were injected with cancer cells. She found results nearly identical to those of her previous study—TT reduced the levels of the same four cytokines. Pretreatment with TT did not matter—the mice still developed tumors, and there was no evidence that TT reduced tumor size. But the results remained the same for the cancerous mice treated with TT as in the first study—cytokine levels were reduced and tumor migration inhibited, suggesting her initial finding was not a one-off.

I could not understand why scientific colleagues in the integrative oncology community were not paying attention to the groundbreaking research with cells and animals in this field. Although I knew that as a Jain who did not believe in harming animals I would not personally engage in such research, I understood that the Western world would find placebo-controlled animal research compelling to help answer the age-old mechanism questions and move beyond the "energy healing is just a placebo" skepticism. Certainly, many scientists would say that if the results Gronowicz and the Harvard researchers reported were compelling, we should find studies from other labs and perhaps discover whether biofield healing has promising effects for our immune systems.

BIOFIELD HEALING AND CANCER: SYNERGISTIC DISCOVERIES

I dug deeper and learned more about the history of healing experiments on animals with cancer. These positive findings on biofield therapies affecting cancer outcomes in mice were not limited to the use of TT. Bill Bengston has been researching the effects of biofield healing on cancer for decades and developed the Bengston Method, which he has taught to many people, including skeptical scientists.[9] Through years of conducting studies on mice with cancer in collaboration with different universities, Bengston reported that mice injected with lethal amounts of cancer cells (that should have died as a result) lived when they were treated with biofield therapy.[10] Paradoxically, however, he found that although the mice receiving biofield therapy did not die or seem sick, their tumors were still growing. Bengston describes his findings: "The mice treated with 'healing with intent' techniques typically developed an encrusted blackened area on the surface of the tumor, followed by tumor ulceration, implosion, and then full lifespan cure. No mice went into remission spontaneously without receiving a healing treatment."[11]

Bengston reported that in several experiments, even though the mice did not seem sick, animal ethics committees expressed concern because the tumors in the mice kept growing. Often the research team was told to euthanize the mice before the experiments were complete because of the tumor sizes.

Margaret Moga at Indiana University was curious about the Bengston Method. She devised a study to look more deeply at the biofield therapy by having Bengston send healing energy to the mice in the same room and do the same from a distance. Moga found that overall, for mice with small tumors (< 120 millimeters) treated by Bengston, seven of ten had complete remissions. However, for the mice with larger tumors (> 120 millimeters), none of the eight mice showed complete tumor remission.[12] The study team suspected immune changes were somehow involved, but in those particular published studies, immune factors weren't specifically examined.

CUTTING-EDGE BIOFIELD HEALING RESEARCH AT MD ANDERSON CANCER CENTER

Most recently, the work examining biofield healing in mice with cancer has been taken up by Lorenzo Cohen, a psychoneuroimmunology researcher and longtime colleague in integrative medicine. Cohen is a distinguished professor of clinical cancer prevention and director of the Integrative Medicine Program at the University of Texas MD Anderson Cancer Center, where he has been serving for more than two decades. When I was conducting my study with fatigued breast cancer survivors, Cohen contacted me to learn more about my work. At that time, he was already receiving large grants from the NIH and National Cancer Institute for clinical studies in acupuncture, expressive writing, and Tibetan yoga. However, he was also deeply interested in biofield healing work because he had experienced energy himself as a young child.

Cohen shared that his grandmother, Vanda Scaravelli, a tremendous influence on him, was a yoga master who trained with B. K. S. Iyengar. She would play with her grandchildren by grounding herself energetically so that no matter how much each of them tried over the years, they simply could not lift her. Even two adults could not pick up this petite woman weighing 100 pounds. Later, as a scientist and dedicated yoga practitioner, Cohen would still wonder: How did that work? Like me, he understood on an experiential and theoretical level that energy, or the biofield, was present not just for healers but was likely a driving force in the health benefits of meditation, qigong, and yoga. Cohen was determined to get the scientific community closer to understanding a mechanism for biofield effects—or at least how energy directly influenced physiological pathways in cancer research.

Cohen became acquainted with Sean Harribance, a healer tested by several labs for his psychic abilities and brain activity correlations with these abilities.[13] Harribance and Cohen began talking about possible studies on biofield healing. The time of the biofield center grants had passed, and as I have mentioned earlier, NIH was simply not interested in funding further studies in biofield science. Initially, a private donor showed interest in backing Cohen when he wanted to study Harribance and determine whether technology could replicate the biofield healing effects the healer might demonstrate. As with many healers, the proposal to develop technology based on his abilities was concerning to Harribance. He questioned the overall intent of such studies, worried about maintaining his intellectual property rights, and was skeptical about device development. Harribance was more interested in exploring the science behind the effects he was seeing.

After years of delicate communications and cultivating the highest integrity for the work with his colleagues at MD Anderson, the funder, and Harribance, Cohen convinced all parties to commence the research with the agreement that the focus would be on pure science, not device development. They followed other studies' lead by looking at Harribance's ability to heal both human and mouse cancer cells in a dish, along with cancer cells in mice, using non-small-cell lung carcinoma cells (NSCLA 549, a type of lung cancer in humans) and Lewis lung-cell carcinoma (a type of lung cancer in mice). The research team examined whether Harribance's emitted energy, compared with sham healing, influenced cancer cell growth, related immune cell function, and other pathways. Harribance treated the animals with five sessions for thirty minutes each over three weeks.

As you read this book, the research is still going on, and the initial results are, again, profound. Cohen and his colleagues at MD Anderson Cancer Center somewhat replicated what the Harvard researchers found with Yan Xin, the qigong healer. When Harribance practiced biofield therapy on the human lung cancer cells in a dish, the researchers found reduction in the cancer cell proliferation and downregulation of the protein kinase Akt—the same protein kinase found to downregulate during the Harvard studies when treated with qigong energy emission.[14] The results suggest that both types of biofield healing are influencing a critical molecular pathway that helps to promote cancer cell death (apoptosis). The researchers also found that mice treated by Harribance showed reductions in tumor size and that this was related to reductions in the inflammatory cytokines interleukin-6 and tumor necrosis factor.

The MD Anderson Cancer Center researchers also found other important immune changes related to reducing cancer cell growth and decreasing the tumor's ability to protect itself. Cohen and his colleagues found that the chemokine monocyte chemoattractant protein-1 (MCP-1) related to increased cell growth and migration of lung and other types of cancer was also reduced in the mice receiving Harribance's therapy. They also found twofold increases in white blood cells associated with killing tumors (CD8+ cytotoxic T-cells) in the mice Harribance treated, along with downregulation of programmed death ligand-1 (PD-L1), a protein expressed on cancer cells. This protein helps to form a biochemical shield that protects tumor cells from being destroyed by the immune system. PD-L1 is one of the downregulation targets for novel immunotherapies that have transformed the cancer treatment landscape, resulting in cures never seen in the history of oncology. But in this study, it wasn't a novel immunotherapy that downregulated the PD-L1 in cancer cells in mice—it was Harribance's healing ability.

Also completely striking but not mentioned in the first scientific publication was how the mice responded to Harribance when he came to their cage. Essentially, the mice knew right away when he arrived and tried to get as close to him as possible. Whenever he came to the cage, even if he wasn't giving a healing treatment, the mice would crowd right at the front of the cage as if they were expecting something good. Cohen was curious about this and explored whether the mice would do the same if a man of similar size came to the cage. The mice wouldn't crowd for anyone else— just for Harribance—showing that creatures we might assume have less consciousness than humans are more perceptive than we think. The mice might have sensed energy associated with Harribance and the healing effects they were receiving. (Honestly, my heart breaks when I think about these mice—crowding to the front of the cage for his healing energy to help rid themselves of the cancer with which they were injected.) Cohen shared the full story, as well as a video of Harribance and the mice, with me during a Consciousness and Healing Initiative (CHI) webinar—if you're interested, you can find it on our webinars page at chi.is.

Like any good researchers, the scientists at MD Anderson Cancer Center attempted to replicate their initial research and determine whether they could drill down further into cellular mechanisms to understand how biofield therapies were driving these changes in tumors. This time, replicating the experiment with the same type of mouse lung cancer, they didn't find reductions in tumor size with biofield therapy as they had found in the first study. What they did find was similar to Bengston's results. Mice treated by Harribance had a significant and substantial increase in death of tumor tissue (necrosis). The tumor cells had ulcerated, as Bengston had reported in his study. When the MD Anderson Cancer Center researchers looked at the exposed tumor tissue, they found that mice treated with biofield therapy had 2.3 times more cleaved caspase 3 positive cells (markers for cell apoptosis) than in the control tumor tissue. The researchers also found replications of changes in specific cell subsets related to antitumor immunity, as they had found in their first study. They also found that the mice treated by Harribance were "calmer," as indexed by their behavioral activity, with 50 percent less time spent in frantic movement compared with the activity of the sham treatment control group mice.

What's next for these researchers? Given the groundbreaking nature of this work—showing that a biofield healer can reliably alter tumor physiology toward profound change—I've wondered why Cohen has been publishing this research in more niche integrative cancer journals rather than mainstream science and medicine journals. Cohen informed me that it is not for lack of trying. The more mainstream medical journals are not yet interested—but, Cohen hopes, with greater use of controls, pharmacological blocking of pathways that suggest further cellular mechanisms are causing the effects, measuring and blocking the emissions from the biofield therapies, and clearly determining the mechanisms of action, mainstream scientific and medical journals will take more notice of the work.

I've recently connected Cohen with Bengston because I was surprised that they had not been fully aware of each other's work. I've also connected both of them with a foundation that will be funding their and others' research. There will be a fruitful line of research with biofield therapies on mice at MD Anderson Cancer Center—and, I hope, with humans.

REIKI TREATMENT FOR STRESSED RATS

Exploring the biological effects of biofield healing in animals has gone beyond cancer. Ann Baldwin, a professor in physiology at the University of Arizona, has conducted a study on Reiki healers' effects on immune function in rats. Baldwin, another mainstream researcher turned biofield healing enthusiast, was introduced to Reiki by her postdoctoral student Meera Jain. Jain knew of Baldwin's work investigating the effects of noise stress on rats in labs. Studies had shown that noise caused significant enough stress in these caged rats to induce inflammation—particularly leaky gut—and Jain noticed that not all the investigators were aware of these effects.[15] Jain was a Reiki master and wondered if Reiki might help reduce this stress in these lab rats and whether they might experience changes in immunity as a result. Baldwin didn't know anything about Reiki at the time, but Jain convinced her to do a study and helped write a grant funded by the NIH in the early 2000s to conduct the research.

Baldwin's researchers studied four groups of lab rats. One group received no noise, another received noise, another received noise and Reiki, and another received noise and sham Reiki. They found that rats exposed to noise showed increases in inflammation as measured by microvascular leakage in their guts. However, rats who received Reiki showed a significant decrease in this stress-induced leakage. The rats receiving mock Reiki did not experience a decrease in this stress-induced leakage.[16] Having witnessed these effects of Reiki on her rats, Baldwin learned more about Reiki. She became a Reiki practitioner herself and published several other studies looking at Reiki's effects on practitioners, patients, and even more rats—examining other physiological effects such as heart rate.[17]

PUTTING IT ALL TOGETHER: WHAT THESE CELL AND ANIMAL STUDIES SAY ABOUT HEALING

If your mind is whirling from all the data these researchers found, let me summarize the key points:

- In the past decade alone, at least four different investigators at three different universities and a prestigious medical center in the United States (Harvard University, Indiana University, the University of Connecticut, and the MD Anderson Cancer Center), all using biofield therapies and sham control treatments, have reported that different types of energy healing can affect tumor growth, tumor death, tumor migration, and related cellular immune function in different types of cancer in both animal and cell culture studies.[18]

- Several studies in independent labs have shown evidence for some intelligence in these biofield therapy effects—specifically, that they influence cancer cells and regular cells differently and that they influence protein kinase pathways related to cell growth differently depending on whether the cells are cancerous or not.[19]

- These cancer studies examined different types of biofield therapies, not just one type, and most assessed effects of extraordinary healers. Based on studies so far, it's still unclear just how much experience you have to have as a biofield healer to influence these types of effects or what the optimal dose of energy healing might be.

- Effects of biofield therapies on cell function and immune response have also been demonstrated for normal cells and animals, not just for cancerous conditions.[20] Importantly, not all results have been replicated.[21]

These studies help us to know that biofield therapies can't be fully understood by relegating them to placebo effects. These studies suggest that biofield healing affects our immune system intelligently and materially in cancerous cells while not having such effects in normal cells. These initial studies show synergistic effects on immune and cellular pathways. They tell us that the energy transmitted through healers affects our immune systems all the way down to cell signaling—in ways we are only beginning to understand.

How is this happening?

As you can imagine, scientists want to know the mechanism of biofield healing. Although I honestly question whether trying to identify a singular mechanism for energy healing makes sense, it does make sense to attempt to understand how this kind of healing has these profound effects. Let's explore some theories on biofield healing mechanisms in chapter 9.

CHAPTER 9

What's the "Mechanism" for Biofield Healing?

Given that we've learned that biofield, or energy, healing has significant and substantial effects that cannot be explained solely by placebo effects on patients with cancer, pain, and other ailments—what then, is the mechanism by which this healing might work?

This question has been a thorn in the side of many biofield researchers. Even when effects of healing emerge, many mainstream medical journals refuse to publish the findings because the mechanism is unknown. Funding agencies such as the National Institutes of Health (NIH) have stated that in order to grow the science behind biofield therapies, a "plausible biological mechanism" must be proposed and tested first. This might seem like an unreasonable barrier to the study of biofield science. After all, we don't know how all drugs or devices work—even though we might find one mechanism of action, we might find later that a drug or device works in a different way than we previously discovered. (This is part of the reason so many drugs have off-label uses—we think the drug acts on specific neurochemical pathways and then find out later it also works on other pathways related to other diseases.)

We might also wonder: Aren't clinically significant effects of biofield therapies on patients, combined with a high benefit-to-harm ratio, enough to warrant a deeper look at integrating these therapies in medicine, even if we don't know the mechanisms? Finally, what if the mechanisms are nonphysical in nature and cannot be measured? Despite these points, it's become clear that in the material world of science and medicine, understanding the mechanism on a physical level is important to scaling up biofield research.

As you might imagine, theories by scientists and healers abound as to how biofield therapies work. Both research and practice perspectives are crucial for us to understand how biofield therapies have profound healing effects. Let's look at a few different explanations of the mechanism of energy healing and explore where current evidence supports or refutes these ideas.

THEORY 1: BIOFIELD THERAPY RESULTS ARE JUST PLACEBO EFFECTS

Haven't we ruled out this explanation? Yes, in a way we have, but the answer also depends on what we call a *placebo*. As we've explored both in this and the previous chapter with clinical studies on biofield therapies, the data show they have more effects than placebo or sham controls both on psychological functioning and on immune system changes to a statistically significant extent. But we can't say that what we call a *placebo element* doesn't actually have effects. In other words, if all living beings have a biofield, then placebo elements such as positive therapeutic interactions (fueled, for example, by feelings of empathy, love, and connection) might actually shift the biofield between the healer and the client—and alter the patient's physiology. The energy of our emotional state, or our "vibes," might be felt by others and influence their physiology without us even talking to them. Thus, what might be considered a placebo effect—positive therapeutic interaction—might actually reflect biofield changes.

Kathi Kemper's study at the University of Ohio is an example of how emotions "sent" by one person can be felt by another person—without the recipient even knowing about the practitioner's intention. In her carefully controlled study, Kemper found that a skilled meditator who sent lovingkindness to another person in the room, even without the subject knowing it was happening, shifted the recipient's heart rate variability (a measure of heart health) in a positive direction—toward greater parasympathetic nervous system (rest-and-digest) activity.[1] Therapists are often taught to hold a space of unconditional positive regard for patients during psychotherapy—and unconditional positive regard in itself has been shown to have significant healing effects on patients.[2] Kemper's study begs the question: What is the difference between sending love and sending healing? Is it a placebo effect, is it a biofield effect, or is it both?

As I discussed in chapter 5, studies show that placebo elements—such as expectations, conditioning, relationship, and ritual—all have profound effects on our biology, down to our cells healing. These elements are present in every therapeutic encounter. As I suggested in chapter 5, placebo elements, from a biofield and consciousness-based perspective, can be reframed as Holistic Elements Activating Lifeforce (HEAL). To some degree, HEAL is present in every healing encounter, including biofield therapy. Instead of trying to subtract them from any clinical research model and trying to prove these therapies are "better" than placebos, perhaps we should be considering how clinical therapies (including biofield therapies) augment HEAL so that we can empower our own healing no matter what type of therapy or medicine we choose.

THEORY 2: BIOFIELD THERAPIES' EFFECTS ON BIOLOGY CAN BE EXPLAINED BY LOW-LEVEL ELECTROMAGNETIC FIELDS (EMFS) THAT AFFECT BIOLOGICAL "RECEPTOR SYSTEMS"

Basic science already teaches us that our bodies, down to our cells, give off low-level electromagnetic fields (EMFs).[3] Our cells also emit low-level light particles known as biophotons.[4] We are currently exploring what these energy emanations from our bodies and cells tell us about our state of health.[5] In fact, researchers using biofield devices are exploring how we can measure the human energy field as well as alter our biology and improve health by using certain frequencies of energy.

Although different aspects of every human biofield can be measured, the main question is whether healing practitioners demonstrate specific, reliable shifts in electromagnetic energy related to healing effects that might explain the changes in cellular function we see with biofield healing. The other big question is whether human bodies have specific receptors sensitive to these biofield effects that propagate changes in body physiology.[6]

Could it be that one mechanism is a healer's unique signature of an electromagnetic field affecting biological changes in another person? Are there biofield receptors in our bodies that translate subtle energetic signals into positive biological changes? Although this concept might seem farfetched to some scientists, emerging evidence from different fields of medical study such as bioelectromagnetics, molecular biology, regenerative medicine, and pathology, taken as a whole, suggests that (1) EMFs might play a role in biofield healing, and (2) receptor systems exist in the human body:

- *Different researchers have reported finding EMF emanations from healers during their healing practices.* These include measurable changes in brainwaves and brain activity, direct current fluctuations and biophoton emissions from their hands, and magnetic field changes.[7] However, not all healing practitioners have demonstrated these results, and it's unclear how reliable these changes are even for the healers studied.[8]

- *There is evidence that both healers and EMF devices affect cell signaling, cell growth, and healing of bone cells and cancer cells.* In the studies I mentioned in chapter 8, biofield therapy has affected cell growth, signaling, and functions in different cell types, including bone and cancer cells. Several EMF devices have shown effects on cell signaling and healing, including in bone cells and cancer cells.[9] However, no studies to date have examined healers and devices side by side, using the exact same model in the same experiment, to see if the effects on cells are the same or different.

- *There appear to be "biofield receptors" on DNA that respond to low-level electromagnetic changes, affecting gene transcription.* As with biofield therapy research, studies examining precise mechanisms for EMF device effects are in early stages. However, at least two promising studies have shown that low-level EMFs (< 300 Hz) can alter gene expression by activating specific promoter regions of DNA called *electromagnetic field response elements* (EMREs).[10] Researchers at Columbia University have theorized that these parts of DNA might be responsive to EMFs by conducting electrons in DNA.[11] This research field is still small, and again, no studies have compared potential effects of healers and devices on gene transcription and influences on EMREs.

- *Evidence suggests that biofield healers and EMF devices might affect the same cellular pathways.* More than twenty studies have shown that EMFs affect voltage-gated calcium channels and that EMF effects on biology can be inhibited by drugs that block those calcium channels.[12] One study from Georgetown University has also shown that biofield healing increased intracellular calcium in a cell culture model and that this effect was mediated by changes in voltage-gated calcium channels. As in studies on EMF, blocking the voltage-gated calcium channel suppressed the effects of biofield therapy on increasing intracellular calcium.[13] However, this is only one study with no independent replication, and again, no comparisons of healers with EMF devices using the same model have been made.

Collagen and the Interstitium: A Possible Bodywide Receptor System for Biofield Effects

EMFs and biofield healers' energy might also propagate "bodywide" through connective tissue.[14] Healing practitioners who say they can feel or "see" energy in the body when they work have often stated that they sense energy moving down fascia, or connective tissue, organized in a whole-body network just below the skin. What does the science say?

Helene Langevin, a longtime acupuncture researcher and currently the director of NIH's National Center for Complementary and Integrative Health (NCCIH), reported an 80 percent correspondence between acupuncture points and connective tissue planes.[15] She and others have also reported that collagen bands (collagen is the fibrous protein structure found in connective tissue) have lower electrical impedance (i.e., less electrical resistance, or more current flow). In some cases, connective tissue planes corresponding to acupuncture meridians have shown lower impedance compared with areas of connective tissue not associated with these meridians—however, the data are mixed, and more studies should be conducted.[16]

Why would there be lower electrical impedance (i.e., greater current flow) in connective tissue planes? We are learning more about these planes and how they might connect the organs. In 2018, Neil Thiese (a New York University professor of pathology with expertise in the liver and a scientific advisor at the Consciousness and Healing Initiative [CHI]) and his colleagues published a groundbreaking study reporting the discovery of a new, bodywide organ (like the skin is a bodywide organ) called the *human interstitium*. The interstitium is a network of fluid-filled pockets between our cells supported by a network of collagen bundles. This matrix of collagen bundles interspersed with fluid is connected all over our body, from our skin to our muscles to our digestive system to our bladder, and the fluid empties into our lymph system through the lymph capillaries.

Collagen fibers, like all protein structures, are charged molecules—that is, they have and carry electricity. Collagen fibers in the interstitium are physiologically active and might interact with cells as they travel through the fluid matrix, which consists mainly of water. The water in the interstitium likely serves as a way electrical charge can propagate through the collagen network. The late scientist Mae-Wan Ho described the phenomenon of charge conduction through collagen, noting how bound water layers on the collagen fibers likely provide proton conduction pathways for rapid signaling throughout the body.[17] It's important to understand that this matrix of fluid in the interstitium is highly organized and dynamic, with several different kinds of cells (including integrins, desmosomes, hemidesmosomes, connexins, etc.) that can and do interact with each other to foster changes in immunity and healing. For example, interactions between these matrix cells help cells such as fibroblasts, osteoblasts, and epithelial cells to move to certain areas of the body where they are needed. Longtime biofield researcher and colleague James Oschman, author of *Energy Medicine: The Scientific Basis*, was proposing effects of biofield healing on what he calls the *living matrix* for decades—well before studies discovered the bodywide interstitium.[18]

It might come as no surprise, then, that scientists are calling for more research into this newly found anatomical structure, noting that it might help us better understand cancer pathology as well as effects of acupuncture and movement therapies.[19] For example, it could be that movement (including stretching, tai-chi, and yoga) or the stimulation of acupuncture needles activates the bundles of charged collagen in the interstitium. From there, these activated fibers can influence the flow and activity of cells that travel across the interstitium, affecting immunity.

Could the interstitium really be part of the explanation for biofield therapy effects on the body? Perhaps, but we would need to understand how the "charge" of energy healers is getting through the skin because, in this case, there is no movement of the connective tissue or needling of the tissue. We also need to understand how at least some healing practitioners seem to be emitting measurable amounts of electromagnetic current. Could part of the answer be in our skin itself?

Merkel cells are a unique class of sensory receptor cells located in the inner part (basal layer) of the epidermis (outer layer of skin) in humans as well as other mammals. They are connected to the dermis, the inner supportive layer held together by collagen, where much of the body's water supply is stored. (Merkel cells, considered part of the epidermal-dermal junction, are specifically connected to the dermis via hemidesmosomes.[20]) Merkel cells are sensitive to light touch as well as to EMFs.[21] Interestingly, these cells are not distributed uniformly—for example, there are more Merkel cells near the fingertips.

Merkel cells contain pigment granules composed of neuromelanin, an iron-containing magnetic material. In the presence of a magnetic field, the melanin-containing granules, called melanosomes, move and activate the cells in a process called mechano-transduction. Merkel cells are also neuroendocrine cells, meaning that when activated, they produce hormones. They also collect in "touch spots" in the skin that connect with nerve fibers that send information to the brain.

Merkel cells are already known to activate sensory neural pathways.[22] Could it be that the activation of Merkel cells in response to a subtle charge (such as low-level EMFs) triggers the nearby connective tissue in the dermis? It is plausible that biologically generated fields from healing practitioners might activate Merkel cells in the recipient. The Merkel cells in the recipient could then activate sensory neuron pathways and influence immunity via collagen pathways in the interstitium. This is not a new idea—the involvement of Merkel cells in human biofield sensing has been proposed before but has not been explored scientifically.[23]

Despite controlled studies showing that biofield healers have effects on biology, we are far from understanding how healing "gets under the skin."

I am presenting pieces of a puzzle that has yet to be put together. If we want to find out how energy gets under the skin, we're going to need a serious program of research that, at the outset, includes biofield scientists along with scientists in microbiology, biophysics, neuroscience, bioelectromagnetics, immunology, fluid mechanics, and dermatology. And even then, an understanding of how biofield healing might be electromagnetically, mechanically, and chemically transduced under the skin to influence our cells might not explain the full picture of healing.

THEORY 3: BIOFIELD EFFECTS ARE NONLOCAL AND NONLINEAR AND MIGHT BE MORE LIKE "INFORMATION" THAN "ENERGY" EFFECTS

Saying that biofield healing effects only result from EMFs is problematic for several reasons. First, not all healing practitioners who have effects on cells and humans have had measurable EMFs. Second, it's not clear whether the healers who have shown measurable EMFs demonstrate exactly the same EMF signature every time they heal someone. Third, no studies have yet related EMF emanations from a healer directly to biological changes in a recipient. And fourth, and possibly most important, explaining these effects as electrical current can't necessarily account for the data from distant healing. Numerous controlled studies show that distant healing and intention of distant healers show effects on biology—in animals, cells, and humans. So how does that part of biofield healing work? It can't be "energy" as most physicists describe it.

By definition, *energy* is the capacity to do work. EMFs, the way we currently understand them in classical physics, are said to drop in intensity with distance. We can calculate this. If biofield healing effects were only classical EMF-defined energy effects, then there should be absolutely no effect of distant healing at all. This is why distant healing drives everyone crazy—it doesn't fit our concepts of energy. To explain how distant healing works, we have to explore other physics models beyond the classical model. Yes, we might have to go quantum here.

I'll admit it. Even in my early days as a student, whenever someone would invoke quantum physics as an explanation of energy healing, I would roll my eyes. I couldn't help it. But to be honest, I didn't understand it. We were never taught about quantum physics in our biology or neuroscience classes—or in our immunology classes. Back then quantum physics was theory, or at least it was shown only to be an effective explanation for miniscule phenomena such as how quarks (smaller than atoms) behave with each other. So how do quantum physics principles help explain real biological changes in healing practices? As it turns out, quantum physics and its application to biology might not be as woo woo as some thought. Why?

First, we now know from quantum physics experiments that nonlocal information transfer via entanglement can and does happen in macroscopic and biological systems. *Entanglement* is where two objects, seemingly separate, are actually interconnected in ways we can predict and measure (by measuring their spin, for example). These two (or more) entangled objects form an interdependent system, considered *nonlocal* because influencing one part of the system influences the other part(s) even if the parts are far away from each other. You might have heard this described by Albert Einstein as "spooky action at a distance."

Scientists have known for a while that entanglement isn't just found between subatomic particles. Entanglement, which many people might consider an abstract concept, has now been shown—in carefully executed physics studies published in the best scientific journals in the world by different groups—to apply to macroscopic objects, even solid structures, and even to biological systems behavior in animals, cells, and plants.[24] Discoveries in macroscopic entanglement have actually formed the basis for technology such as quantum computing.

It makes one wonder: If our minds can conceive of and create quantum information transfer between computer chips, could human beings ourselves function like the quantum computers we have created?

So how does entanglement work? A study published in 2001 in the prestigious journal *Nature* reported the entanglement of two macroscopic objects (gas cesium atoms) separated in space. The scientists connected these atoms using a pulse of coherent light that created an entangled spin state between them (i.e., the light pulse influenced the two cesium atoms, separated by long distance, to spin together in a complementary way). These and other early studies demonstrated the principle of quantum nonlocality and showed how light can drive information transfer between macroscopic parts of an entangled system. This paved the way for what was called *quantum teleportation*.[25]

Whoa, wait—quantum teleportation? That sounds like *Star Trek*. Well, not quite—although the fact that some scientists recently reported the groundbreaking discovery of a photon's quantum teleportation on Earth to another photon on a satellite about 1,400 kilometers away got people excited about being "beamed up."[26] Let's be clear here—the photon didn't get physically beamed up. What did happen is that the information from the photon on Earth got transferred to the photon about 1,400 kilometers away.

This is not science fiction—quantum mechanical experiments such as these and others have shown that this quantum information transfer can happen between macroscopic objects in a profound manner. In fact, a study published in *Nature* in 2017 examining entanglement using a photon in a crystal demonstrated that this photon of light entangled more than two hundred macroscopic ensembles of atoms. What's more, each of these ensembles are subsystems with a billion atoms—and showed entanglement all the way down to each atom from this one individual photon. This multiparty entanglement demonstrated that one single excitation—caused by one photon of light—can share information across not just one but many interconnected systems—and in a solid structure.

Entanglement doesn't happen just with atoms and crystals—it happens in biological systems. Scientists are exploring entanglement, as well as other quantum mechanical phenomena such as coherence and tunneling, to explain biological processes and behavior in living organisms—including in photosynthesis, enzyme activity, olfaction (our sense of smell), and magnetoreception (sensing EMFs).[27] Quantum fluctuations in the brain have even been proposed as a necessary link to understanding consciousness. More than twenty years ago, for example, Stuart Hameroff, a professor of anesthesiology at the University of Arizona, proposed the idea that quantum wave collapse in microtubules in the brain could explain human consciousness.[28]

Entanglement might even play a role in understanding natural animal behavior. For example, research from different labs suggests that entangled electrons present in birds' eyes help them "read" the Earth's EMF to navigate flight.[29] There is also reported entanglement-like behavior in fish.[30]

CONSCIOUSNESS, ENTANGLEMENT, AND HEALING

You might wonder how consciousness fits into the picture here. After all, several theorists and scientists relate the principles of quantum mechanics to the nature of consciousness, including the relationship of quantum mechanics principles with the Vedic perspective on consciousness.[31] How might this relate to healing?

The supposition is that quantum physics not only informs us about the nature of consciousness itself but also it informs us of universal laws that apply to biology as well as other fields. For example, physicist Menas Kafatos, endowed professor of computational physics at Chapman University, proposes that quantum principles of recursiveness (think "as above, so below"), complementarity (seemingly opposite things that actually unite), and creative interactivity (dynamic systems interaction) are fundamental laws of the universe and laws of consciousness that apply to biology.[32] Thus, the quantum-like behavior we see even in animals and plants is not surprising. However, understanding how nonlocal healing happens might entail a collapse of the quantum wave function in a manner that influences a biological system. That is, in order to understand distant healing effects on biological outcomes, we would have to trace how the information seemingly shared nonlocally influences a biological receptor that triggers a local physiological response.

These are all provocative data and interesting ideas—and yet I would be remiss if I used these data to tell you we have proved that quantum entanglement is how distant healing works. These experiments aren't on distant healing and don't directly test entanglement as an explanation for distant healing. There are many gaps in the data that would need to be filled. Even if quantum physics is the most satisfying theory to explain distant healing at this point, there are many questions to answer, such as: Precisely how does the role of the conscious observer(s) influence or shift the entanglement effects? What determines the strength and duration of entanglement, and how would resonance effects influence that?[33] Are there really just a few types of receptors that might translate this information into meaningful biological signals, or are there many? As tempting as it is to say quantum entanglement is the answer to understanding distant healing on the physical level, we are far from having the precise experimental data to definitively explain the physics of distant healing.

However, the point here is to share with you that what we have been led to believe for so many years by mainstream science and medicine—that we are separate, unconnected beings who don't transfer meaningful information to each other—is simply not true. We have seen this fallacy of separateness in medicine when we thought our bodies were made of separate organ systems that didn't talk to each other. Discoveries in psychoneuroimmunology and other fields help us understand how interconnected our organ systems are and how those interconnections matter for our health.

The quantum physics experiments take this even further to help us understand that even if we are separated in space, we are not separate from each other. Nonlocal information exchange across space between bodies is real and actually happens—both in the lab and in nature. Information transfer is not just a phenomenon observed in biofield healing.

So the appropriate equations and experiments for understanding the precise physics of how distant healing works remain to be seen. However, if quantum physics shows us that we are deeply interconnected across space and even time, then distant healing, just like these multitudes of quantum teleportation experiments, is not an anomaly—it's part of universal law.[34]

SO THEN . . . WHAT'S THE MECHANISM FOR HEALING?

I've just presented at least three possible explanations of how biofield healing works, and there are many more. Here is the problem, from my point of view.

We seem to think we have to pick one of these and leave the others behind as if they don't matter and as if they don't help explain the data. And we're basically taught that until we can completely refute the most mainstream theory, we shouldn't even be looking for explanations for the "inexplicable." This is, from my point of view, the conundrum of solely using Occam's razor for consciousness and biofield research at this point in time. Occam's razor is a philosophy (some might say "dogma") that the correct way of doing science is to follow the law of "parsimony," or explain effects as simply as possible, while refuting other explanations that might be more complex and therefore unnecessary (think "simple is beautiful"). This is the way all scientists are taught to engage in research, and for good reason. We don't need to create new, complex theories or create new laws to explain things that likely follow basic, tried-and-true scientific laws. But sometimes, in our zealousness for parsimony and in keeping with current worldviews, we throw the baby out with the bathwater and turn away from systems-based thinking, even if it is better at explaining all the data.[35]

Let's take healing as our specific example here. If controlled studies on distant healing and positive intention are showing actual physiological effects, and quantum mechanics experiments are supporting theories of nonlocal information transfer—does that mean we throw quantum mechanics out the window as an explanation or pretend that distant healing doesn't exist because we can still explain some healing effects through EMF signaling or even what we call *placebo effects*, which are more parsimonious (simple) explanations? Or, conversely, even if we can experimentally show that some aspects of healing are nonlocal, does that mean local effects such as therapeutic interaction and setting don't matter even if we know they facilitate and augment a healing response?

What I am proposing here, and throughout this book, is that instead of engaging in either/or, or separatist, thinking, we need to move to both/and, or inclusive, systems thinking—particularly as we reach to understand phenomena such as consciousness, healing, and biofield science. (Honestly, inclusive systems thinking is really a solution for remedying all the polarizing situations in which we find ourselves now, not just in science and medicine.)

For example, we know placebo effects are real, we know EMFs seem to play a role in physical healing, we know distant healing and intention have real effects on biology, and we know quantum mechanics experiments support the idea of nonlocal information transfer. What if all of these things are simultaneously true?

If we give up the idea that we have to choose one mechanism, we can still develop robust, testable, and fairly simple theoretical systems-based models of healing that help us understand all of the data, as opposed to ignoring some data because it doesn't fit the current way we've been taught to think.

Currently, we could compile the information from (1) first-person observations reported by healers, (2) ancient theories based in first-person observations from those who have explored the depths of consciousness over millennia, and (3) all the experimental studies in clinical, preclinical, and distant healing to surmise that *healing effects are multidimensional and comprise nonlocal (information transfer) components and local (energetic and physiological transfer) components*. This would hold whether healers are in the same room with the recipient or whether they are in different locations. After all, there appears to be a nonlocal component even when healers and recipients are in the same room—as evidenced by healers' and patients' reports of experiencing the presence of ancestors or guides during healing, for example. There is also a local component of downstream bioenergetic, physiological communication shifts in the body that occur during healing, even if healing is happening from a distance. And, there are local effects of therapeutic interaction and physical environment that play a role in healing.

We need to look at healing from a full-spectrum, whole-person, systems-based approach, with outcomes that relate to patients' experiences as well as possible changes in the biofield during healing. As healing affects consciousness along with emotional, interpersonal, mental, and physical functioning, it is important that we examine a broader range of outcomes to understand the depths and processes of healing.

For example, scientists at the Institute of Noetic Sciences recently examined the effects of extraordinary healers on reducing carpal tunnel pain. This novel study not only reported that healing provided reductions in pain and changes in heart rate variability for patients but also that structural changes in water occurred after healing.[36] The study also incorporated a qualitative component by having a "seer" (a reported clairvoyant) reporting her perceptions of changes in energy fluctuations during the healing. (One of the investigators, Helene Wahbeh, shared the results of this published research in a CHI webinar—you can find it on our webinars page at chi.is.)[37]

These data all help us to understand the different ways healing—whether of ourselves or others—happens. Placebo effects are real, biofield healing is real, and entanglement is real. But the real question is what role you want these discoveries to play in your own healing.

HEALING BEGINS WITH US

As the Jain nun wisely said to me at the beginning of my healing inquiry, the most important approach we can all take is to realize our full healing potential. It really doesn't matter whether we think the effects result from quantum entanglement, energy, a placebo, the brain, or just plain connection with God or nature. If there is one takeaway I hope you will buy into, it's that you have tremendous power to heal yourself and others if you choose. And, by the way, by saying that, I'm not saying that you shouldn't ever take physical medicine. Remember, we are thinking both/and, not either/or. We can refuse to engage in polarizing thinking by exploring possibilities as synergistic instead of antagonistic. We are simply readying ourselves for the best healing response possible by bringing our own consciousness and biofields into the picture for full-spectrum healing. We are on the road to becoming sovereign healing agents who have tremendous power to shape our own health and lives.

To aid you in your healing journey, I've provided a consciousness-based guide to healing in part III using simple, tried-and-true practices that can and will work with any healing path you choose for yourself. These healing keys integrate much of what we've learned about the power of self-healing—some of the strongest healing principles and practices from scientific evidence alongside biofield-based wisdom practices from time-honored spiritual traditions—so that you can engage in your own full-spectrum healing and experience yourself as the free, blissful being you are meant to be and truly are.

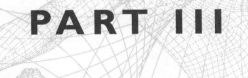

PART III

The Healing Keys—with Exercises and Meditations

The most important thing we can do to integrate the science of healing and the wisdom practices of spiritual traditions is to put our own healing into practice. To help us do that, I've integrated the best of evidence-based practices as well as powerful bioenergetic and spiritual practices into real-life healing keys. These are tools for healing that aid us through our multifaceted and sometimes unpredictable lives. You don't have to go on a ten-day or even weekend retreat to unlock these keys. You can simply do them to aid you in your healing process as you go along in daily life.

As you explore these exercises, you'll notice major positive changes in your abilities to heal yourself, deepen your well-being, and shape your life according to your desires. In each chapter, I've shared some data to help you understand the relevance of each of the keys to your healing process. I've shared some stories as well to give you a sense of how I came to realize the power of these healing keys for myself.

You'll find these keys helpful whether you are new to healing or whether you're a seasoned practitioner. There are different practices and perspectives to match you where you are. Some of the teachings and exercises draw from clinical psychology and behavioral medicine, and some are more esoteric and spiritual in nature. Some are basic practices, and some are advanced. I encourage you to begin the basic practices and then explore the advanced ones as and when you see fit.

Remember that your path of healing is not an either/or. Healing is not antimedicine in any way. Every single healing principle and practice I've shared here works, whether you choose herbs, psychotherapy, drugs, surgery, or vaccinations, for example. If you and your doctor find these approaches medically necessary, there is no conflict with you continuing to heal yourself from the emotional, energetic, interpersonal, physical, and spiritual levels as well. You can still use the keys I've provided no matter what medicines you choose to take. The healing keys are simply bringing your soul's force back into powerful alignment with you so that whatever you need to harmonize in your body, your mind, and your life can occur with greater ease and impact.

For this part of the book, I recommend that you go stepwise from chapter to chapter because each chapter builds on the previous one. You'll begin to see how these healing keys work together in a way that makes you feel fully alive and full of joy and healing power. Enjoy!

CHAPTER 10

Ground for Health

For most of my life, I've never been one to pay attention to my body. You know the famous line by James Joyce, "Mr. Duffy lived a short distance from his body"? That was definitely me, as a typical academic who lived in my head. Having children gave me a newfound respect for my body and the wonders of what it could do. But my motivation to explore what it means to be fully in and feel all sensations in my physical body (embodiment) as well as what it feels like to be connected with the Earth (grounding) came from a discussion with my healing teacher, Reverend Rosalyn Bruyere. I was stunned the first time I heard her and her husband and coteacher, Ken Weintrub, stress the importance of exercise for healers. "Exercise?" I inquired. "Why?"

"Healing," said Rosalyn, peering at each of us intensely, "is a *physical skill*. You've got to know how to ground and develop your physical strength to be able to run energy. I lift weights every day."

She was right. I shouldn't have been so shocked, given all the research about the power of exercise for improving health, such as decreasing inflammation, reducing risk of cardiovascular disease, and improving mood and sleep. But I was floored to notice a difference so quickly. Within a few weeks of lifting weights just half an hour for a few days a week, I noticed that I slept better. I felt stronger and more resilient. My appetite was more regular. I noticed I was much less likely to come down with a cold or flu. My clothes fit better—but most importantly for me, *I felt grounded*. I was aware of more subtle sensations throughout my body and, with that, felt a deeper connection with the Earth as well as my spirit. And I noticed that when doing healing work, what used to feel like a trickle of energy was turning into a more steady flow.

GROUNDING: THE SCIENTIFIC PERSPECTIVE

What is grounding? Grounding is a process of coming into and feeling our physical bodies and deepening our connection with the Earth. Through becoming more embodied and actually paying attention to the feeling of our feet on the ground as well as the sensations in our feet and legs, we allow energy to flow more freely from us to the Earth and the Earth to us. Grounding proponents explain that it works like this: Our Earth, and our bodies, are electromagnetic. As we connect electromagnetically with the Earth, ions from the Earth flow into us, and our ions flow back—reflecting the circulation and interdependence between humans and the Earth that we already know to be true. Grounding opens us up to the bioenergetic level of the body-Earth connection. This is both a subtle energetic practice and a bioelectrical practice. Grounding is a key practice in many traditions, including qigong and tai chi, in which specific exercises are prescribed to foster a deeper connection of our qi with the Earth's qi.

If this sounds like science fiction to you, there is actually research behind the connection between our bodies, the Earth, and even the solar system (though in my opinion, there is much more to explore). Let's briefly dive into some research-based facts to understand the basic relevance of our connection with the Earth.

We have already learned that our bodies are bioelectromagnetic—for example, our bones are piezoelectric—and that our cells emit biophotons that are involved in cellular communication.[1] Not only are we electromagnetic in nature, we can sense the electromagnetic fluctuations in the earth, and these fluctuations can influence our health. Geomagnetic fluctuations not only affect our brains, but also they appear to influence our heart rhythms.[2] Even more striking, these vibratory influences might be coming from beyond the Earth—solar flares, for example, that affect the Earth's geomagnetic field have been found in numerous studies to correlate with heart health, including blood-pressure changes and incidences of heart attacks.[3]

What about grounding in particular? Several studies examined the effects of grounding mats or other devices for electrically connecting us with the Earth. (Think of how you ground your appliances in your home—these devices are doing that for your body—you lie on a mat electrically grounded to the Earth.) Current data from the handful of published studies on grounding have shown improved hormone function, immunity, and muscle recovery, along with decreased depression, fatigue, and pain in adult populations.[4] One study examining grounding with preterm infants reported improvements in heart rate variability—particularly improved vagal nerve functioning, related to the parasympathetic rest-and-digest nervous system, which helps with bodily repair and growth functions.[5]

GROUNDING: THE SPIRITUAL AND BIOENERGETIC PERSPECTIVE

From the ancient biofield and specifically the chakra healing perspective, getting grounded is a way of getting into contact with our *muladhara*, or root, chakra. *Muladhara* means "foundation" or "support"—this chakra is located at the base of the spine. It reminds us of the joy of *being*—there is nothing to do and nothing to feel but simply to be present in our bodies.

In Vedic teachings, muladhara chakra is associated with the Earth element and thus relates to being grounded and connected with the Earth, as reflected by its seed syllable, or *bija* mantra, *lam* (pronounced "luhm"). However, muladhara chakra is also associated with the kundalini energy, described as Shakti, the divine creative feminine force said to lie sleeping or dormant at the base of the spine until awakened. Because of muladhara chakra's connection with the fiery and electrical aspects of kundalini energy, it is also associated with the fire element, as shown by the downward-facing triangle in the visual depiction of this chakra.

Not surprisingly, because of its connection with the Earth and kundalini, the first chakra is strongly associated with vitality as well as the release of karmic patterns, as signified by its Vedic deity (Ganesh, the remover of obstacles and the bringer of joy). The four petals depicted in the image of muladhara chakra speak to the importance of embodiment in experiencing different aspects of consciousness—namely, *manas* ("mind"), *buddhi* ("intellect"), *chitta* ("embodied consciousness"), and *ahamkara* ("ego").

FIGURE 10.1. The first chakra, known as *muladhara* chakra in Vedic and Tantric traditions, means "foundation" or "root." It is connected with the Earth and fire elements and teaches us how to be in our bodies.

THE IMPORTANCE OF GROUNDING AND EMBODIMENT: SPIRITUAL TEACHINGS

Many have taken issue with Vedic teachings of the path toward spiritual liberation in traditions such as Vedanta and Jainism because they emphasize the seeming renunciation of the physical body for spiritual growth. Although it is easy to interpret the texts in this way, another interpretation based on the practices is that transcending the senses does not mean ignoring the body but rather being completely aware of bodily sensations without being attached to them. There is a growing belief in many spiritual traditions that in order to truly transcend the ego and transform consciousness, embodiment is absolutely necessary.

We are comfortable considering our emotions and thoughts as dynamic—perhaps we can even visualize them as more fleeting and vibrational in nature. But many of us have trouble understanding that our body is also a vibration—just a more dense, gross vibration. We might forget that ultimately the body is a physical reflection of the spirit, and that spirit communicates through the body.

Teachings from Vedantic and Jain traditions echo much of what modern-day healers describe: The body is not only a physical reflection of the spirit but also it provides information about all experience. Information is not received simply through floating energy fields. The mind perceives it through the body, much as a speaker transduces electrical audio signals into sound we can hear. If we damage the speaker, we can compromise the sound. As we listen to and take care of our bodies, we open to spiritual wisdom.

Buddhism is perhaps the most popular current tradition that emphasizes the power and value of bodily attention. The practice of Vipassana, often translated as "insight meditation," helps us to see things as they truly are through the practice of carefully observing bodily sensation without attachment or aversion. This practice has often been termed *mindfulness* in the West, and the Western definition of mindfulness as "nonjudgmental, moment-to-moment awareness" certainly describes a core aspect of Vipassana meditation. In Vipassana practices, meditation is anchored in observing bodily sensation. The body serves as an anchor for experience, and the key is not to be caught up in wanting or not wanting the sensations that arise with each experience. We learn to cultivate equanimity toward sensation, and by doing that, we can fully realize and sustain moment-to-moment experience. Because we are anchored in this equanimity, not only can our spirit be in full communication with us but also, eventually, it can be fully liberated.

The good news is that communicating with our spirit and inner guidance is not an all-or-nothing phenomenon. We don't have to be fully enlightened to receive intuitive wisdom. However, the more we are able to feel into our bodies and be comfortable being in them, the more easily we can receive intuitive wisdom.

So, the first steps of any healing process are to get grounded, to be comfortable in our bodies, and to tune in to bodily sensations.

There are many ways to get grounded. As I've mentioned, exercise is one way. Getting into nature is another simple way and is practiced in just about every culture. For example, the *shinrin-yoku*, or "forest bathing," practices in Japan have been studied for their health-promoting effects, and both psychological and physiological health has improved as a result of forest bathing. Specific qigong and yogic exercises help us get grounded. We also just learned about the use of grounding mats.

We can begin our grounding practice very simply by bringing awareness and energy to our lower body. See the following exercise for a bioenergetic practice that we can use to foster a deeper connection with our bodies and with the Earth no matter where we are.

Simple Practice: Getting Grounded in the Lower Body

Here are some simple steps to cultivate groundedness:

1. **Feel your feet.** Whether you're wearing shoes (ideally, your shoes aren't rubber) or have the opportunity to be barefoot (highly recommended), draw your attention to the soles of your feet. In a standing position, try gently bouncing up and down with your legs to help get sensation into your feet and ankles. You can also try squatting a few times to bring stronger sensation into the feet and the legs. Feel your calves, your ankles, and the soles of your feet. Feel as though gravity is pulling you down into the Earth, and feel your feet sinking into the Earth. If you can stand on actual Earth, such as clay, dirt, or sand, that's even better, but even if you're in a high-rise apartment or office, you can still benefit from grounding through your feet. What you are doing is opening the chakras at the soles of your feet. You can also focus your attention at muladhara chakra, at the base of your spine, while doing this exercise.

2. **Breathe in, and release energy out through your feet.** This is really as simple as it sounds. Inhale and breathe in deeply. Feel the air fill your lungs, and open the soles of your feet by keeping your attention there. Direct the flow of your energy downward, and allow your breath and any sense of stagnant or painful energy to flow down your legs, into your feet, and out to the

Earth. You can imagine yourself as a tree with deep roots into the Earth. Allow those energetic roots to really make contact with the Earth, and breathe out into her.

3. **Bring in energy from the Earth, up your legs, and through your lower body.** Now that you've made contact with the Earth, allow the Earth to make full contact with you. Keep the soles of your feet open, and feel the energy of the Earth below your feet. As you inhale, bring the energy of the Earth up through your feet, up your legs, and to your belly. As you inhale, allow yourself to feel it through your lungs while deeply breathing into your belly and solar plexus area.

To be guided by an audio version of grounding meditation, go to shaminijain.com/bookresources.

...

THE BODY AND SPIRITUAL WISDOM

Through my decades of personal practice, research, and teaching, I have come to believe that opening to the wisdom of Spirit within the body is fundamental to living a fulfilled life. The more we make time for this, the more we realize we don't have to force it to fulfill our life purpose or desires. Our body is a vehicle for Spirit, and after we let Spirit in, there is no need for trying. There is no need to seek purpose, for it will find us—and we will recognize what is part of our path and what is not. The first step is to recognize the spiritual wisdom in our body, and learn how to surrender to it.

See the following exercise for a more advanced practice to open the body to spiritual wisdom. It draws from both the Vipassana tradition and the work I have learned from a master healer, my teacher Rosalyn. Give yourself about twenty minutes for this practice.

HEALING OURSELVES

Advanced Practice: Opening to Spirit in the Body

1. First, do the grounding practice as described above. Make sure that you can feel sensation in your feet. As you develop this skill, you will find that you can feel grounded within just a few minutes.

2. Now scan your entire body (you can decide whether you would like to do this lying down, sitting, or standing). From your feet and toes, let your body breathe normally, and while you are breathing, gradually bring your awareness up the body— meaning up your legs, hips, stomach, back, lungs, heart, shoulders, arms, hands, neck, face, back of the head, jaw, sides of the head, ears, eyes, forehead, and top of the head. For this exercise, you are not necessarily focusing on chakras but rather your physical, flesh-and-bone body. You are trying to connect all the way with the consciousness of your cells. See how deeply you can notice sensations in the different areas of your body. After you have gone through your body, just relax and breathe. This should take about ten to fifteen minutes.

3. Come to a sitting position with your back straight. Notice if there is a part of your body clamoring for your attention. (Often unpleasant sensations beg for our attention, but sometimes pleasant ones do as well.) If there is, allow your awareness to rest on that part of your body, and see if you can observe the sensations fully. If any emotions or thoughts come up during observation of the sensations, just make note of them but continue observing the sensations. If there is significant pain or tightness in the area, you can direct your breath to that area of the body if it gives you comfort, but still stay with the sensations. After you feel done with this (I recommend no more than five minutes on this section), move to the next part.

186

4. Bring attention to your heart, and invite Spirit to connect with you through your heart. Spirit, in this case, is whatever sentient, higher power beyond your ordinary self you revere. It might be God by the name you call God, your soul, your innermost self, nature, or the universe, for example. Whomever you call upon, open your heart to receive contact and know that you are safe. Feel free to use a prayer if you are called to do so.

5. Keeping a focus on your heart center, allow yourself to note any sensations you might have during this request for contact. Try to remain here for at least five minutes, quietly, to receive any guidance or wisdom that might occur during this time. Your messages might come through feelings, thoughts, visualizations, or other means. See if you can link the messages with any bodily sensations that might be occurring during your spiritual connection.

6. Give thanks to your spiritual guide, and end your meditation when it feels appropriate for you.

...

The more we deepen our connection with our bodies through grounding, the more we enhance our health and vitality. And, as we allow ourselves to deepen our recognition of the subtle sensations of our bodies and what these sensations are telling us, we realize the full truth of the statement "Your body is your temple." We begin to recognize the signals from Spirit within our body. By cultivating a deeper sense of embodiment for some time, you will begin to recognize, via bodily sensation, when you are getting spiritual guidance to enhance your and others' well-being.

CHAPTER 11

Flow with Emotional Energy

"You just go from zero to a hundred in one second!" sputtered my husband after an outburst about the dishes. "I can't take it!"

The argument was about something all too familiar to couples with young children—dishes. I just can't leave dirty dishes in the sink for the next day—no matter how tired I am. And after we both had put in a full day's work and dealt with two young kids whose greatest form of enjoyment seemed to be doing anything *but* eating their food at dinnertime, our post-dinner cleanup was delayed, and we were both exhausted. Tonight was his turn to do the dishes because I cooked dinner, and I couldn't wait to be done with the evening and relax. I felt my anger rise as we argued about our transactional lives: who did what, when, and how much. Despite knowing better, I just totally lost my cool.

How many of us have felt captive to our emotions? Sometimes it might seem like our emotions run our lives. We've all had times when we've said or done something we wish we hadn't, such as fuss at a child, coworker, friend, or spouse because of feeling angry, anxious, depressed, or just plain overwhelmed.

At the same time, emotions are what provide the flavors of life—sometimes delicate, sometimes bland, and sometimes ever so sweet or spicy. Some might say emotions are what make life worth living. Imagine eating food with no flavor for the rest of your life or listening to music that made you feel nothing. Pretty strange, right? Many would hate to live that way—it would feel inhuman.

But many ancient healers and philosophers said to transcend all emotions for your ultimate well-being. I have read countless books from Hindu and Jain monks and scholars who warned against giving in to emotions and impulses, whether negative or positive, because they saw those as hindrances to the spiritual path and total well-being.

Who's right? As in most cases, both perspectives are right. Emotions are a beautiful part of being human—and at the same time, they don't define us. Emotions are information, and as long as we open to the information and sensations present in emotions and don't dwell in them or try to stuff them away, they can be a huge help to us in our journey to health and well-being.

What do we know about emotions and health? Historically, because we have been more focused on the pathogenic model (i.e., the study of disease), psychoneuroimmunology (PNI) and psychoneuroendocrinology (PNE) have focused on how emotions, particularly negative ones, might worsen disease. However, recently scientists have begun to more deeply research the impact of positive emotions, exploring whether they might even prevent disease. What have we learned so far?

POSITIVE AND NEGATIVE EMOTIONS ARE NOT OPPOSITES

Imagine you are gazing into a beautiful, still lake, and you take a video. You then decide to throw a stone in to see the ripples as they glide upon the lake's surface, and you take another video of the lake, with the moving ripples. Now if you compared the two videos—would you consider the still lake without the stone's ripple effect as being the opposite, or mirror, image of the rippled lake?

At first, you might think the videos are opposite. But if you looked more closely, you'd see that the still lake itself is not really still. It is also ever changing, with water flowing in it in subtle, yet discernable ways. The stillness of the lake is completely relative to the ripples that occurred when you threw the stone. The size and shape of the ripples are determined by the size and weight of the stone you throw. It's the same thing with emotions. Every emotion we feel ripples through our being, whether positive or negative, big or small, and affects us in both subtle and less subtle ways. Although the intensity of the emotion and how long you tend to feel that emotion (i.e., how big the stones are and how often you throw them) appear to make a difference in our health, it seems that positive emotional ripples are not simply the absence of negative emotional ripples. That is, positive and negative emotions are not simply opposite reflections of each other, and even our sense of emotional stillness is relative to our typical emotional state.

EMOTIONS: THE SCIENTIFIC PERSPECTIVE

When we feel negative emotions more often than not over a prolonged period (days and even sometimes weeks), they can lead to what we call a negative mood—a sustained feeling of negativity that often includes anger, anxiety, and sadness. Sometimes we can't even explain exactly what we are feeling—we just know we are feeling "moody." And typically, when we are in that state, we are more likely to blow up or get depressed about events, even if typically we wouldn't react quite that way. The palette of our mood influences the colors of our emotions.

Scientists have discovered that the landscape of negative mood, particularly when colored with frequent experiences of emotions such as anxiety and depression, can make disease progression worse—particularly cancer, chronic pain, diabetes, and heart disease.[1] Whether negative mood over time might actually cause disease is still considered controversial in the medical arena (in part because the types of controlled longitudinal studies needed to confirm whether negative mood or stress cause disease are difficult and expensive to run).

But observational, epidemiological studies with thousands of people and meta-analyses of multiple studies do provide a compelling case about the effects of negative mood on body-mind functioning and disease progression. Here are some highlights:

Clinical levels of depression are associated with greater risk of death as well as risk of developing cardiovascular disease.

Depression predicts increased risk of death in heart failure patients.

Depression symptoms have been associated with increased inflammation in the body.

Some might consider anger a flip-side of depression—and indeed, with anger expressed in a hostile manner, we see similar effects on the body. Those who express anger in a hostile way are more likely to have increased inflammation (and hostile married people might elevate inflammation in their spouses as well).[2]

Hostility is also a predictor of cardiovascular disease risk and mortality.[3]

If negative emotions can drive us toward negative health states, there is good news: We are discovering more and more that a positive mood—such as happiness or joy—seems to buffer or protect us from negative health effects. Current studies indicate the following:

Positive mood is linked to decreased risk of disease, including AIDS, diabetes, and heart disease.[4]

Positive mood might affect health and healing down to epigenetic levels.

Positive mood has been linked to improvements in immunity.[5]

What's more, the effects of positive emotions on health seem independent of negative mood—so, even if we are feeling anxious or depressed, we can still improve our health by having positive emotions.

EMOTIONS: THE ENERGETIC AND SPIRITUAL PERSPECTIVE

When we learn about the effects of emotions on our bodies—particularly the negative health states—we might understand why some of the ascetically minded meditators would prefer to just release the experience of emotions altogether. Who needs that many stones thrown in one's lake?

But emotions can really be our biggest teacher and can be an aid to spiritual growth. The more we are aware, moment to moment, of the subtlety of our emotions, the less they hang around to affect our bodies and minds in more chronic ways. The key, whether it's a pleasant or unpleasant emotion, is to allow yourself to feel it in the moment, learn what it has to teach you, and then be able to let it go.

From the spiritual perspective, most primary emotions—such as anger, happiness, pain, pleasure, and sadness—stem from our basic nature to engage in attachment and avoidance. We like this, and we don't like that. When we experience someone or something we like, we feel a positive emotion, and when we experience someone or something we don't like, we feel a negative emotion. This is the yum/yuck living in which we are all engaged as human beings.

The stickiness occurs when we dwell in our likes and dislikes. For this reason many sages have emphasized the need for detachment—essentially, creating distance from our likes and dislikes so that we can have a wider perspective on the world and more tolerance for all beings that reside in it. This stance would mean we observe our likes and dislikes, but we aren't driven by them. We simply note them as information and allow ourselves to experience our reactions when they come up. It's important to remember that detachment is not repression, and unfortunately, the two often get confused. As it has been said, the only way out is through. When we allow ourselves to feel our emotions, as opposed to trying to get rid of them or clinging to them, we can more clearly hear the messages they bring. Only then can we naturally let go of them.

Modern scientists are finally beginning to understand what spiritual traditions and teachers have been expressing for thousands of years. Our emotions aren't "out there," apart from our bodies. They are connected to and directly influence our bodily functions. From a spiritual perspective, I will share what I have learned from my own work as well as the teachings of Reverend Rosalyn Bruyere to help us better understand how we can work with our emotions on a subtle level, and therefore affect our physical well-being.

EMOTIONS AND THE SACRAL CHAKRA

From a chakra-based perspective, we begin to feel emotions in the *swadhisthana* (second, or sacral) chakra, located near the bladder, in the area of the sexual organs. The sacral chakra, associated with the water element, reflects the fluidity of our emotions and the purity of "life nectar" as well as the process of creative flow—from the beginnings of desire all the way through to birthing and sustaining a new creation (life itself). This chakra also reflects our "first feelings"—the feelings that arise in us almost automatically in response to a situation.

Figure 11.1, a drawing of the sacral chakra from the Vedic and Tantric traditions, depicts a flower with six petals. These petals actually represent *vrittis*, or "whirlpools," of mind disturbance. Each of these petals represents a mind disturbance we are to transcend for our emotional well-being—including unmitigated desire, pitilessness, destructiveness, delusion, disdain, and suspicion. The depiction of this chakra reminds us that access to the purity-of-life nectar and creative force is right here within us. We simply need to clear our mind disturbances to fully tap into this elixir of life—the stillness of water beyond the ripples of emotions. Those of you who practice yoga might have heard of the first line of Patanjali's Yoga Sutras: *Yoga chitta vritti nirodha*. This essentially means the path of yoga ends all disturbances of the mind. By allowing our mind disturbances to settle and cease altogether, we allow access to our true state of consciousness—absolute bliss.

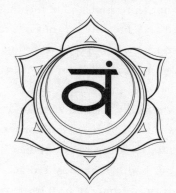

FIGURE 11.1. The second, or sacral, chakra is known as *swadhisthana* chakra in Vedic and Tantric traditions and translates to "one's own abode." This chakra is associated with the element of water and teaches us about emotions, creativity, and life "juice."

When we notice emotions, either positive or negative, we might choose to focus our attention on the bladder and sexual organs, where the sacral chakra resides, and notice the sensations we feel. If we feel strong sensation there, we can choose to work with it in different ways, depending on whether we view those sensations as positive or negative. Being aware of the sensations in our bodies when we have emotions is the first step to emotional freedom and enjoyment.

PUTTING IT INTO PRACTICE
Tuning In to the Body to Notice Emotional States
We might be comfortable fine-tuning our physical bodies with exercise, but we sometimes forget that we need to tune in to our body's inner sensations for our health as well. Bodily sensations provide us with so much information, and being tapped in to the wisdom of the body can help bring our awareness to emotions in order to move through them and let them go. When we tune in to what is happening in our bodies moment to moment, we are more likely to notice our emotional state earlier, manage it better, and prevent it going from zero to a hundred with emotional outbursts. We are able to ride the waves of our emotions in our body and release them more in the moment with ease, preventing the need to unload lots of pent-up emotional energy.

Tuning in to our bodies with breath is a great practice anytime and often even easier to do when we aren't flooded with a particular emotion. The more we pay attention to where our breath is in our body, the more likely we are to catch the energy of a high-powered emotion before it snowballs. See the following exercise for a simple awareness practice to get started.

Awareness Practice: Five-Breath Body Tune-In

Here is a universal, simple practice to foster awareness of your breath and body. You can make this a two-minute or two-hour practice, depending on the time and motivation you have.

1. Focus your attention on the tip of your nose. Notice your breath come in and out of your nose five times. Don't try to change your breath. Just notice the inflow and outflow. Pay attention to the temperature sensations as your breath comes in and out. Is it warmer on the exhale, for example?

2. After you've done this five times, keep watching your breath, but allow yourself to notice where else you feel the breath in your body. Is it more in the chest, or the gut, or throughout your body? Then, notice the quality of your breathing. Is it fast, shallow, or slow?

3. While keeping your attention on the inflow and outflow of your breath, also allow yourself to scan your body. Are there places that feel free and flowing? Are there places that feel painful or tight? Or places you don't feel at all? Just allow yourself to notice what your body is telling you, while keeping connected with your breath.

4. Close the practice by bringing yourself back to your nose and noticing the breath flow in and out of it five more times.

...

I recommend starting this practice when you are feeling fairly neutral, if you can, just to get used to feeling the breath in your body. After you've gotten the hang of the practice, try it when you're feeling a particular emotion.

Notice the ebb and flow of the emotional state in your body, including which areas feel more free and which areas feel more constricted.

Noticing our breathing helps us to anchor into other bodily sensations. After we know where our breath is, we can choose to notice where we are feeling those other sensations. The key right now is just to see how much we can tune in so that we can recognize the vibration that leads to a particular emotion—before we allow ourselves to get caught up entirely in the emotion.

When we begin to recognize the energetic fingerprints of an emotion in the body, we are literally tuning in to the vibration of the emotion inside us and recognizing what vibrations we are putting out to others, even in a subtle way. That information also might help us know what we are feeling before we choose to act—or not act. Bodily awareness is the first key step to mastering our emotions and directing our energy.

REMEMBER TO NAME IT, DON'T CLAIM IT!

As we focus on breathing through our emotions, we will undoubtedly encounter a whole slew of thoughts that accompany our emotions and sensations. We will feel a certain sensation and begin to spiral off on what it means, where it came from, how bad or good it feels, and so on.

Cognitive-behavioral therapy (CBT) often places a lot of focus on identifying behaviors and thoughts that occur during emotions to help us better understand and handle our emotions. Although CBT and other types of psychotherapy have certainly proved useful in treating anxiety and depression, in my view we must go into the body and the biofield, and beyond the realms of conscious thoughts to help resolve the root issues that cause persistent negative emotions and behaviors. Thoughts are tricky—the more you pay attention to them, the more they manifest, and ultimately thoughts associated with strong emotions are arising from the conditioned mind. Getting beyond thoughts allows you to move past the conditioned mind and toward the source of real coherence and real freedom. The simplest way to do that is to stick with your breath.

So when you are breathing through an emotion, recognize your thoughts as helpful information, but don't dwell on them—instead, bring your awareness back to your breathing and bodily sensations as much as possible. You will certainly be aware of thoughts—but just recognize them as information based on patterns of conditioning. Take any insights you might get from the thoughts and move on (unless they are thoughts of harming yourself or someone else—in which case you should immediately find a professional mental health-care provider to help you through the difficult emotions and thoughts). Remember, your thoughts are not the whole of *you*—they are just a reflection of your conditioning.

FOSTERING ENERGY EXCHANGE BY BREATHING INTO DISCOMFORT

After we've begun to tune in to our bodies, we might notice that our breathing changes during emotions, both with negative and positive emotions. During negative emotions, for example, we might notice that our feelings of anger are associated with more rapid, shallow breathing and tightness in certain areas of our body. Sometimes we might realize we are breathing less often and less deeply, almost holding our breath when we feel anxious or fearful. We might notice that some of our negative emotions are also accompanied by unpleasant sensations. These can include a sense of constraint, heat, pain, or even numbness in certain areas. Consider the popular saying about someone or something being a "pain in the neck" (or other body parts!). Those sayings actually stem from feeling bodily sensations in uncomfortable situations—whether consciously or unconsciously.

How do we help to release painful or unpleasant sensations? We foster an energy exchange—literally by breathing into the discomfort.

Why does breathing into areas of discomfort often help shift our state of being? We are literally sending fresh energy, or prana, through the breath to areas that need to loosen up. My teacher Rosalyn is fond of saying, "The solution to pollution is dilution." From a subtle energy standpoint, certain emotions can feel toxic, but they're really just stuck energy of a particular quality, like sticky mud on a shoe. You simply need to wash them off, and some stains are more stubborn than others. To "unstick" ourselves, we simply hose off the shoe with clean water, or in this case fresh, new breath or new energy, to loosen bonds that don't need to stick. Recognize the thought forms sticking to you and keep breathing to let them go.

After you've gotten comfortable with the basic Five-Breath Body Tune-In, you can begin to work with uncomfortable emotions and sensations by simply adding one extra step to foster an energy exchange in areas of discomfort.

The following exercise relates the whole sequence for Breathing into Discomfort:

Breathing into Discomfort Practice

1. Focus your attention on the tip of your nose. Notice the breath come in and out of your nose five times. Don't try to change your breath. Just notice the inflow and outflow.

2. After you've done this five times, keep watching your breath, but allow yourself to notice where else you feel the breath in your body. Is it more in the chest, or the gut, or throughout the body? Then, notice the quality of the breathing. Is it fast, shallow, or slow?

3. While keeping your attention on the inflow and outflow of breath, also allow yourself to scan your body. Are there places that feel free and flowing? Are there places that feel painful or tight? Are there places in the body that you just can't feel? Just allow yourself to notice your body while keeping connected with your breath.

4. Now allow yourself to send fresh breath in a loving way to any areas of discomfort. Allow yourself to feel the sensations of discomfort while also feeling as though your breath is like fresh water, able to loosen any solidity of sensation that you might

feel and dissolve any felt blockages or pain. You might have reflections or realizations as the discomfort begins to move. Just take note of them, but keep your attention on your breath, and continue to breathe into areas of discomfort. Allow your breath to touch uncomfortable sensations and wash them away as if by a clean stream of water, down your legs and into the ground. Do this for five full breaths.

5. If the discomfort feels intolerable, feel free to move your attention to a part of your body that feels neutral or even pleasant. Rest in those sensations, and whenever you feel ready to go back to breathe into discomfort, you can begin again.

6. Close the practice by bringing yourself back to your nose and noticing the breath flow in and out of it five more times.

...

If you had particular realizations as you were breathing through the discomfort, write them down in a journal or notebook. What was your uncomfortable emotion or sensation trying to tell you?

When beginning to breathe into discomfort, I recommend starting slowly and letting your body guide you. Try it for five breaths at first. Focus simply on sending the breath to areas of your body that you think need it, and let your thoughts wander as they do, always coming back to the breath when a thought leads you here or there.

Don't worry if the unpleasant sensations don't completely resolve. They might even feel more unpleasant at first while you are directing more attention to them. After you begin breathing into discomfort, you might become more aware of unpleasant sensations, such as heat, pain, stinging, or tightness. You might connect more deeply with an emotion like anger or sadness. Whatever you are feeling while breathing into the discomfort, allow yourself to feel it. Gradually you'll notice that if you don't stuff the feeling but just breathe into it, it will dissolve over time. As everything is in constant flux, so too are our emotions and sensations. Sometimes the process takes time. If you feel like you've hit a geyser of emotion, allow yourself the space and time to simply breathe through it. It might not resolve immediately, and that's okay.

If you are feeling significant sensations of anger or pain, remember to allow any intense sensation you are feeling to flow down and out the bottom of your legs. Feel as though you are releasing the sensations into the Earth. You are literally grounding yourself and releasing the energy of anger and pain when you do this, allowing for fresh energy from the Earth and from your breath to replenish you. If you have feelings of sadness, allow yourself to release it through crying or whatever process feels right, but keep breathing through the emotions. Sadness can be particularly draining, so it's important to keep nourishing your heart and your self with fresh energy through your breath. At the end of this process, beyond the release of sadness, you might even feel the energy of self-love.

FOSTERING POSITIVE EMOTIONS

Of course, we are not just beings seething with negative emotions to release, nor do we want to be! Although positive emotions are not just opposite reflections of negative emotions, it is also true that one way to pull ourselves out of a negative funk is to do things that make us feel good. As we learned, positive emotions can also be considered preventative medicine—the more positive we feel, the more resilient we are during stress and the resulting health issues.

What's more, positive emotions themselves are contagious, so when you're being positive yourself, you're helping someone else be positive as well. Perhaps you've had the experience of feeling better yourself after being around someone in a good mood! Practicing positivity and generating positive emotions are truly the most important individual and social health practices you can do.

Here are some science-based, practical tips for fostering greater positive emotions:

1. **Do something you generally *love* to do (even if you don't love it right now).** The research is pretty clear on this. Behavioral activation—that is, allowing ourselves to do something we enjoy—really helps our mood, down to helping combat clinical depression.[6] Motivating yourself to do something you generally love, even if you don't think you'll love it now, appears to be totally worth it. Doing something you love helps ignite your passions— "lighting your fire" and bringing you "joy juice." From the esoteric energy perspective, doing something physical is associated with our first chakra, our "power battery," which fuels our life energy and will to live. Pleasurable feelings work with the second chakra, the source of creative energy. So when we physically engage in something we enjoy—whether it's hiking, playing a sport, singing, or taking a walk with a friend—we are building new life and creative energy, allowing stuck energy to move through us. That fresh energy brings us into a clearer, more creative, and joyful state. We learn to nurture ourselves and celebrate our passions and joys, which we can then choose to share with others. If you're feeling down, you might not feel motivated to do much at all, even things you used to enjoy before. This is all the more reason you should allow yourself the possibility to experience joy—even if you're not sure you will feel any differently. With a bit of effort, you will remember and reconnect with that joyful part of yourself and recognize how the flow of emotions is ever changing—meaning that even when we are feeling depressed, "this, too, shall pass."

2. **Get creative.** We greatly underestimate the power of creativity to foster positivity, connection, and well-being in our society. Consider the connections between creativity and emotions. We can use our creativity to express our emotional state beyond words, to deeply communicate our state with others, and even to break through our state of conditioned consciousness. By the very nature of your being alive and human, you are a creative being. You might not consider yourself creative if you aren't an artist,

dancer, musician, or poet by profession. But that same creative spark you might admire in others is present within you. The more you express yourself creatively, the more you cultivate pure energy you can harness for any purpose you choose. Your creative act doesn't have to be a magnum opus—a fancy, big production—it can be as simple as singing your favorite song in the car, putting together a fun outfit that expresses your feelings that day, or enjoying experimenting with cooking a new meal. All of these activities tap into the second chakra energy through and beyond your emotional state and free up your energy to foster growth and vitality. Because I feel creativity is so incredibly vital (pardon the pun) to our well-being, I've dedicated chapter 12 to creativity and authentic expression—so if exploring creativity is new to you, don't worry. Chapter 12 will get you motivated to see the links between creativity and happiness for yourself!

3. **Foster and spread networks of happiness.** Is happiness really contagious? A recent large-scale study suggests that your happiness is not just influenced by those you're in direct contact with but also might extend up to three degrees of separation—meaning that you're more likely to be happy if your friend's friend's friend is happy.[7] Although that might seem unbelievable, if you consider the strong evidence of links between social connection and happiness, and the ability to communicate our emotions through conversations and behavior, including even social media—it begins to make sense. Speaking of social media, you will likely not be surprised that a recent study has confirmed what many of us have suspected—that Facebook posts with positive or negative emotional content actually influence the spread of similar posts, suggesting that our emotions are influenced by the information we take in through social media, and we continue to spread the content that we receive.[8] This all points to the power of our networks in helping to establish and spread our positive emotions—and means that your sharing of your own positivity might in fact lift up someone else! Following are

some suggestions for increasing your happiness network.

4. **Reach out and schedule time for a positive connection.** Connect with your positivity network! It doesn't matter if it's a family member, a friend, a pet, or your favorite tree! Just allow yourself to be absorbed in another being's positive energy for a while—whether in person, by phone, or by video chat. You might feel compelled to share your own joy (or your sorrow). But having that heart-to-heart with someone who cares and who generally makes you feel good can make a world of difference. Do this regularly if at all possible—particularly if you are feeling lonely.

5. **Pay positivity forward.** This is as simple as it seems. Do something that forwards the happiness of another (without compromising your integrity, of course), and you will increase your happiness in the process. One study reported that those who volunteered to help others reported increased happiness—regardless of whether they had high or low socioeconomic status.[9] This makes sense from a consciousness-based point of view. When we choose to help others, we are on some level recognizing that we are not separate from them. Our desire to help others is not separate from our desire to help ourselves—we can see ourselves in those people. Thus, doing something to uplift another will naturally allow us to feel uplifted as well because we are dipping into a consciousness beyond our conditioned self.

As we begin to explore the realm of creativity, positivity, and positive emotional energy, we begin to realize that a big part of our health and well-being is also about the ability to express ourselves in a way that honors who we are and how we're feeling. Let's explore the role of authenticity and self-expression in your well-being in chapter 12.

CHAPTER 12

Express Your Creativity to Jump-Start Vitality

Have you ever felt like you lost a part of yourself?

Sometimes it happens. Life changes, and we change with it. It could be a move, job change, marriage, kids, taking care of elders, or any sort of transition. Sometimes it's not even a difficult transition that makes us lose a part of ourselves but a decision we make to keep on with some things and release the rest. And yet, we might regret leaving that part of us behind. Often, the part of ourselves we leave behind is a creative part of ourselves that we might think, in today's world, is less important or less valued.

This certainly happened to me—for about fifteen years. Basically, I lost my voice. As much as I loved singing, for reasons I could not fully understand, I knew part of my path was to continue in my study of healing. Unfortunately, when I chose graduate school, I also decided there was no point in singing anymore if I was not "serious." Not only did I relinquish my opportunity to prepare for a professional career in classical western opera singing—I simply stopped singing altogether. And by making that black-and-white decision, based more in perfectionism than in feeding my heart and soul, I lost a huge part of myself for more than fifteen years. Singing was a gift I was given to bring me back to my own creative bliss—

but I had been blind to its purpose for most of my life. And a part of me literally felt like I had died.

I'll bet many of you can relate. External circumstances seem to shift the tides of our lives so that sometimes we lose parts of ourselves society doesn't necessarily directly reward. If we enjoyed art, dance, music, or other areas of creative expression when we were young, unless we pursued these passions as professional artists, we might have lost sight of them over the years. We often think we have to leave creative pursuits behind in our process of "adulting"—making money, providing for a family, and pursuing a career. However, losing that creative juice comes with real costs—we can end up losing our ability to innovate, our fluidity, and a great deal of our joy.

Thankfully, our creativity is never really lost. In my case, I found the joy of singing again spontaneously while singing to my kids when they were young. When they got a bit older, I decided to reclaim the fun of singing for myself. Out of the blue, I created a Guns N' Roses cover band called Nuns N Moses. I searched for musicians and convinced them (all straight males) to dress as nuns while I dressed as Moses for part of the show, changing lyrics and singing songs from Moses's perspective. It was hilarious fun while paying homage to one of my favorite childhood rock 'n' roll bands with excellent musicians. Soon after, I was asked to front an Iron Maiden tribute band called Up the Irons. The music was amazing, and the band was a hit, with thousands of fans and a busy gig schedule at the best venues in Southern California. I found myself blissfully singing my heart out—and I had more energy than I ever had in my life.

I share this personal story with you for two reasons. One is to remind you that the parts of you that you think are forgotten actually live on inside of you—particularly the creative parts of you. These are the parts that long for authentic expression, in whatever ways they are able to manifest. They do not die, and when we give them voice, we actually provide healing for ourselves—an ability to bring us to a greater sense of self-awareness, self-expression, connection, and ultimately transcendence. The second reason is to challenge you to consider ways you can step out into a more authentic expression of yourself—even if it feels risky to you. The best thing you can do is to break the false idol of yourself. Creative expression gives you the tools to connect with yourself beyond your cultural and social conditioning and to connect with others in true heart and soul expression. Nothing can be more freeing and more healing.

CREATIVITY, HEALTH, AND WELL-BEING

Often when we think of creativity, we think of the arts, although creative expression can take many forms. Still, much research explores the impact of creativity on health outcomes by examining how engaging in art therapies such as dance, expressive writing, music, and visual art affects patients' physiological and psychological health. A comprehensive review of studies reports that music therapy (which includes listening to music as well as, in some cases, improvising music) has been found to reduce anxiety and stress and improve hormone and immune function in a variety of patients, including those with cancer, coronary artery disease, and other health issues. Studies with dance movement therapy report similar outcomes: It reduces anxiety and depression, improves body image, and increases positive emotions.[1]

Expressing ourselves through art therapy is also healing. Studies have shown that patients with cancer, chronic illness, and trauma who engage in art therapy (including drawing and painting) report decreases in anxiety and stress and improvements in well-being, including self-worth and sense of purpose. The healing effects of creating and expressing can also be in the form of words as well as pictures—dozens of controlled studies in expressive writing (writing about our emotions or simply free writing) have shown that expressive writing leads to decreases in fatigue and pain as well as improvements in immunity and mood.[2]

How do these therapies heal us down to our cells? There is growing interest in the neuroscience of creativity. However, we have more questions than answers around the precise neural mechanisms involved in creativity.[3] The psychoneuroimmunological model has been highlighted as an area for further research.[4] Following are some important takeaways from the studies I mentioned above:

1. **Creativity in any form matters.** There are so many ways to be creative, and the research suggests that whatever avenue of creative expression and cultivation we choose, we will likely see benefits in terms of well-being and positive bodily health effects. Creativity

is not just defined by the arts—it refers to the ability to generate new or novel ideas; thus, creativity can be experienced on the emotional, mental, physical, and spiritual levels in different ways.

2. **Creativity boosts confidence.** The data suggest that engaging in creativity, whether privately or in public, can increase our self-acceptance, give us a stronger sense of mastery, and in some cases help us to express ourselves more clearly and authentically to others.[5] Cultivating these qualities of environmental mastery and self-acceptance has health benefits in and of itself—studies have shown that women with higher levels of environmental mastery and self-acceptance have, for example, less depression, better insulin resistance, and even improved sleep.[6]

3. **Creativity is an everyday process.** A final takeaway from the research is quite profound. It suggests that the best way to enjoy the benefits of creativity for well-being is to continue being creative and enjoy everyday creativity. Some studies suggest that if we stop engaging in our creative expression, we might start to see the loss of benefits on our mood. At the same time, research reports that on days when we are more creative than usual, we tend to generate more positive emotions the next day.[7] Creativity is a continuous process of self-expression and evolution, so, as with formal spiritual practice, the more regularly we engage in creative acts, the more benefit we might see. We also need to convert the relationship between our belief that we are creative beings and can be creative to actually being creative and receiving the benefits. Studies are clear that the more we believe in our ability to be creative (sometimes called creative self-efficacy), the more likely we are to reap its benefits, which include improved work performance.[8] When you accept and express your own creativity, you also begin to notice and appreciate creative expression in others—from the food they make to the clothes they wear to the way they express themselves in their bodily movements. I now recognize that we are all creative beings, expressing ourselves

in diverse ways. After we align with the creative force within us, we gain energy through positive emotions, which help us to persevere through difficulties and also experience life with more joy.

CREATIVITY: THE SPIRITUAL AND BIOENERGETIC PERSPECTIVE

The relationships between creativity, sensuality, sexuality, and vitality have been noted in ancient cultures across the world.[9] Interestingly, even Western academic researchers have described creativity as "spiritualizing the passions."[10] From the spiritual and bioenergetic perspective, it is no accident that creativity is linked to both emotional health and vitality—in fact, from the chakra healing point of view, there is a deep connection between creativity, emotional energy, and sensuality, including access to states of bliss.

Creativity is often associated with the second, or sacral, chakra, located in the area of the sexual organs (see figure 12.1). The second chakra's Sanskrit name is *swadhisthana chakra*, loosely translated as "one's own abode." The second chakra is associated with the element of water, which corresponds with cohesion, flow, fluidity, life, and purity. All these qualities relate to creativity, emotions, sensuality, and sexuality. Working with the second chakra is where we can jump-start our own creative energy—which, frankly, is powerful enough to create life itself. In Taoist tradition, the area around the second chakra is known to hold what has been described as "essential energy," or life essence (*ching qi* or *jing qi*, generally described in women as residing in the ovaries).

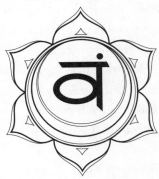

FIGURE 12.1. The *swadhisthana,* or second, chakra in the Vedic and Tantric systems. This chakra is associated with creativity, emotions, and flow.

PUTTING CREATIVITY INTO PRACTICE
Fostering Our Flow

How do we begin to jump-start our experience of creativity and its links to flow, improved mood, and vitality to augment our own deeper, more authentic expression of ourselves and our healing? Following is an easy guide:

1. **First, recognize that you are a creative being.** The more you identify yourself as a creator, the easier it will be for you to create in different settings, even at work. Even the scientific data suggest this.

2. **Start simple.** Remember that no one defines what is creative except you. Is there a particular creative activity that draws you to it? It does not matter whether you have prior experience with it. It does not need to be a specific art form, either (putting creative outfits together or improvising a meal without a recipe are examples). Pick something easy for you to engage in at least once a week for six weeks, and do something that you can easily fit into your day or week. (Singing in the car or dancing around the house for fifteen minutes a day counts!)

3. **Go beyond judgment.** Suspend your and others' judgment, and move beyond your discomfort. Believe me, I know what it's like when the kids beg you to stop singing in the car! You will encounter a whole slew of judgmental statements, most of them likely from yourself. As Nike loves to say, "Just Do It." (In my case, when encountering my children's complaints, I keep singing, but I do it more softly so as not to irritate their eardrums beyond belief.) When feeling uncomfortable, do it anyway and tap into the bodily, energetic feeling that you have when you are being creative. That will help you break through those negative self-judgments and clear those *vrittis*, or mind disturbances!

4. **Observe, persist, and enjoy.** Notice how you feel after engaging in your creative act. Be your own scientist. Explore how you feel

after the first time, and then the second time, and so on. How did the rest of your day go after you allowed yourself some time for creativity? Keep at it, and even try your hand at something new. You might feel more comfortable working with an art form you have learned in the past. However, remember that your goal is not perfection—it is connecting with the energy of creativity. There is something to be said for examining an art form with "beginner's mind." Keep honing your creativity by focusing on both things you know and things you don't know, and see what insights come to you as a result.

To help you actualize these guidelines, I've included a Fostering My Creative Flow Worksheet at the end of this chapter. Use this for your exploration into creative, authentic expression to foster your healing and vitality.

And now that we've learned how to ground, flow with emotions, and get authentically creative to foster a stronger base of energy and vitality through our bodies, we're ready to begin to put that positive energy to good, directed use for our healing. Let's explore in chapter 13 how to use the science and practice of intention and ritual to focus and power up our healing process.

Fostering My Creative Flow Worksheet

CREATIVITY SELF-REFLECTION

When do you consider yourself most creative?

_____

_____

_____

_____

What is a creative act you can feel comfortable committing to do on a regular basis?

_____

_____

_____

_____

When do you feel the most flow in your body?

_____

_____

_____

_____

When do you feel the most joy?

_____

_____

_____

_____

HONORING MY CREATIVITY—COMMITMENT
(Commit to something that feels like it will be enjoyable and easily doable for you!)

To spark the seed of creativity, vitality, and health, I commit to deeply connecting with my creative flow by _____

_____

for a time period of _____ minutes, at least _____ times per week.

HONORING MY CREATIVITY: NOTICING THE EFFECTS
As soon as you can after engaging in your creative act, note how you feel below. Write in your own words as you see fit, and focus on your emotions as well as your bodily feelings/sensations. Do this for each time you engage in the creative act (ideally at least over a six-week period).

Week 1:

_____

_____

_____

_____

_____

Week 2:

_____

_____

_____

_____

_____

Week 3:

Week 4:

Week 5:

Week 6:

...

CHAPTER 13

Set Your Healing Intention
Through Ritual

Now that we've learned how to ground and cultivate greater energy and allow it to flow, with emotional awareness and creativity, we can begin to shape this energy toward a specific intention we might have for our own healing.

Recall from the chapters in part I that healing is multidimensional and essentially refers to the restoration of harmony—whether on the emotional, energetic, interpersonal, mental, physical, or spiritual level. This can be within ourselves, between us and someone else, or even in the relationship between ourselves and the larger world. Because our world is constantly changing and moving—and we're moving with it—we are always in a process of restoring balance and harmony.

In other words, healing isn't static, and as we discussed earlier, it isn't just about clearing out a disease—although that might happen. Healing is a process, not an outcome. So whether you have a diagnosis or not, healing is always an opportunity to lead you back toward your essential nature, pure consciousness, with its qualities of oneness, truth, and bliss. Healing intention carries you through your healing journey day to day.

In this chapter, you'll first begin to get intimately acquainted with your healing intention and carry it forward with energy to manifest that intention.

The intention might end up being for you personally, whether healing for a specific disease, emotional or mental state, or your general well-being. You might intend healing for someone else who asked for help. You might even find that the intention coming through is to foster healing for our society or the world (clearly, we can use more of that). You'll learn more about your healing intention and set your healing volition, or will, to carry out healing through healing ritual.

INTENTION, EXPECTATION, AND RITUAL: THE SCIENTIFIC PERSPECTIVE

The scientific research does not explore healing intention as much as it explores the effects of healing attention and expectations for health outcomes. Healing attention in this case refers to the practitioner-patient relationship, which we'll explore more in chapter 14, on connection. For now, let's consider the links between healing intention and expectations.

In research, intention itself is more difficult to operationalize and measure because it might be conscious or unconscious. But the downstream effect of healing intention—the conscious expectation of whether a treatment will help—is easier to measure and is reflective of intention. Recall our discussion in chapter 5, in which we found that expectations are key placebo elements that reflect conscious choice-making about whether we feel a treatment is bound to help us. Our consciously communicated treatment expectations (which we can note in a survey question for research) reflect our healing intention. As we become more conscious of our healing intention, we can more readily shape our expectations, which in turn shape our experience of reality.

In terms of expectations, the good news is that whether your doctor fosters your positive expectations for healing or whether you have positive expectations on your own, the data clearly show that your own positive expectation of healing will improve your health. Consider the following evidence:

A recent systematic review of twenty-five randomized studies reports that when physicians enhance patients' healing expectations by providing positive information about the illness or the treatment, patients' health outcomes improve.[1]

A recent systematic review of sixteen studies examined the effects of expectations on recovery for patients with a variety of conditions, including alcoholism, heart attack, heart surgery, hip fracture, hysterectomy, and more. The authors reported that in fifteen of the sixteen studies, patients who had positive expectations about their recovery process had significantly better health outcomes. This included less need for painkillers, greater abstinence from addictive substances, quicker ability to move after surgery, greater weight loss, and better psychological outcomes.[2]

Positive expectations not only drive our health outcomes when we are in a recovery phase from an illness or injury but also they improve healing from more chronic issues such as anxiety, depression, and pain.[3]

Placebo research also shows that just by our expecting a benefit from treatment (even when there is no drug), we reduce our pain considerably, at a clinically significant level. This has been found for patients with chronic pain, idiopathic pain, migraine, and osteoarthritis of the knee, for example.[4]

Expectations affect us down to our neurotransmitters. For example, positive expectations for pain relief, even when no active treatments are given, appear to stimulate our body's own painkillers (endogenous opioids) to release and thereby relieve our pain.[5]

Positive expectations about our healing also influence areas of our brain (including the anterior cingulate and lateral orbitofrontal cortex) involved in how we process emotions and thinking and how we experience pain.[6]

You might be wondering: If expectation can have such powerful effects, why can't we simply expect to be healed and therefore heal? Why do expectations seem to work for some people or at some times and not others? Perhaps you have had the experience yourself of feeling like you had positive expectations for your healing process, and you weren't trying to fool yourself—you really believed it—but it simply didn't happen. Why do expectations not seem to work all of the time?

HEALING EXPECTATIONS AND INTENTION: SPIRITUAL AND BIOENERGETIC PERSPECTIVES

I believe our healing expectations might not work all the time because sometimes our conscious expectations of healing might not be fully aligned with the energy from our true healing desires or with a strong will to carry out our healing intentions (including adopting health behaviors that will aid our healing).

Desires are not always known to our conscious, waking mind. In fact, many desires generally reside in the subconscious, where they might be bound up with or even buried under old memories, patterns, or thoughts actually clouding the energetic power of our desires to carry out our will for healing. Biofield therapy practitioners often note how emotional energy can get "stuck" in the biofield, preventing its free flow throughout a person's system. This description by healers bears similarities to Jain descriptions of consciousness and the biofield, which I shared in part I. These teachings suggest that our karmic impressions, sometimes called *samskaras*, shape the emanation of our soul's energy, thereby affecting our biofields and resulting behaviors and thoughts.[7]

In other words, the pure healing light from our inner selves, our "regenerative energy," if you will, can go only as far as we can allow it. If our biofields are filled with mental afflictions, including anxiety, disbelief in our own power, poor health habits, or trauma, we are essentially blocking that regenerative energy from having its full effect to carry out our healing intentions.

Put another way, healing expectations are mental constructions. Mental constructions have no power of their own—they must be married with the energies of desire and volition (the power to carry out one's will) to actually shape reality. This relates to what ancient Tibetan and other philosophies described as the necessary marriage between the mind and the vital force. In Vedic terminology, this process is often referred to as creating a *sankalpa* (pronounced "SUN-kulpuh"). Sankalpa has been loosely translated into "intention" in English, or sometimes "resolution," but it is multilayered in its meaning as well as deep in its process.[8] In Sanskrit, *san* refers to connecting with our highest truth, and *kalpa* refers to a vow.

Creating a sankalpa is the process of going within to first discover the true desire of the inner heart, bring this desire to consciousness, and then surrender to the outcome most aligned with our soul's growth and purpose. We connect the vital force with this inner desire, with the stillness and depths of consciousness and the resolve of the mind, to give power and shape to intention, and then surrender to it.

KEY CHAKRAS IN SETTING HEALING INTENTION

To fully form a sankalpa, we can work with all of our energy centers. However, two chakras are key to consider in terms of how they help to manifest our intentions: *manipura chakra* (the solar plexus chakra) and *anahata chakra* (the heart chakra).

We'll explore each of these chakras and their relevance to intention—but first an important note: Everything you learned in the previous few chapters leads up to this. The energies of muladhara chakra (the first chakra) and swadhisthana chakra (the second chakra) are essential for connecting with and manifesting intentions. It is important we understand that no single chakra is working in isolation.

To manifest healing intentions into physical reality, we need to be grounded and running strong and clear energy. This is why the foundation of our healing process includes first connecting with the Earth and getting enough energy to be present in our bodies (chapter 10), second seeing and freeing ourselves from negative emotional patterns that bind our energy (chapter 11), and third allowing ourselves to creatively express who we are and how we feel to allow a greater flow of energy within us (chapter 12). These relate to the energies of the first chakra (Earth) and second chakra (water). The more we feel grounded in our lower body, feeling the solidity of the Earth in our body as well as the fluidity of our energy, the more we can use that energy to aid in clarifying and making manifest our intentions.

When we allow ourselves to experience these fundamental human rights—to be in our bodies, to feel what we feel, and to express ourselves creatively—we build energy and skill to release mental-emotional-energetic blocks and open to bring in new energy that guides us toward our next steps. It's a constant process because we are constantly responding to the world around us as well as releasing energy from the past.

MANIPURA CHAKRA: BALANCE, CLARITY, AND INTENTION

As we bring our awareness from our grounded state and fluid sense of self up the body, we encounter manipura chakra, translated as "city of jewels," the third chakra in Vedic tradition (see figure 13.1). This brilliant chakra is associated with the element of fire, but some healers (including my teacher, Reverend Rosalyn Bruyere) relate it to the air element. This is particularly interesting given the clarifying nature of this chakra. Rosalyn describes how we move from "I am" (first chakra, where we are grounded in our life force) to "I feel" (second chakra, where we begin to feel the fluidity of our feelings) to "I think" (third chakra, where we begin to perceive and express). Both the fire and air elements of manipura chakra help us clarify our desires, clear what is not needed, and better express our intentions.

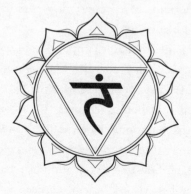

FIGURE 13.1. *Manipura* chakra, the "city of jewels," is the third chakra in Vedic and Tantric traditions. It is associated with the elements of fire and air and teaches us how to clarify and balance our thoughts and carry out desired action.

This is part of your personal alchemy—now, with an awareness of who you are and how you feel (first and second chakras), with the fire and air energies of manipura (third chakra), you are burning away the dross of what doesn't serve you (prior conditioning) and airing out impurities (including all the "shoulds," "should nots," and "ought tos")—to behold the jewels of your own true desire.

Manipura chakra not only helps us to clarify and express what we think, but also it helps us to collect and keep our energies in balance for action. In the yogic system, manipura chakra is where subtle energy currents converge. Specifically, *prana vayu* (an upward-moving current of subtle energy) and *apana vayu* (a downward-moving current of subtle energy) are said to meet in manipura chakra, and particular yogic pranayama exercises aid in this meeting of powerful currents.[9] When we bring these energies into harmony in our bodies, we feel stable, centered, and empowered to bring forth committed action.

Thus, manipura chakra aids us in setting intentions by first helping us clarify our desires with clearer perception and a strong will. We are then ready to move to anahata chakra, the heart chakra, to aid in deepening our intention for greater cocreative power.

ANAHATA CHAKRA: EXPANDING INTENTIONAL CONSCIOUSNESS

Anahata chakra is the fourth, or heart, chakra in the Vedic system. *Anahata* refers to "unstruck sound," and it is where the soul resides and where deeper levels of consciousness begin to be accessed. The description of this chakra relates to the four levels of sound described in Vedic tradition, relevant for manifesting intentions within different layers of consciousness.

The grossest, or most physical, level of sound, *vaikari*, is the actual sound made by our vocal cords rubbing together, for example. The next subtle level, *madhyama*, is considered to be at the kinesthetic-subtle vibrational level, where we might feel sensations or subtle vibrations in our bodies associated with a particular sound, mantra, or even thought. The next, even more subtle level of sound is called *pashyanti*, often experienced more as light than sound. Finally, the most subtle and all-encompassing level of sound is called *para*—Oneness itself. This is beyond our concepts of amplitude and frequency; it is Being itself and can be considered the nature of our soul.[10] This description of the all-encompassing Oneness from which all manifestation is brought is explained in many other spiritual traditions as well. For example, the first sentence in the Gospel of John from the Christian tradition starts with "In the beginning, was the Word, and the Word was with God, and God was the Word."[11]

How exactly do these levels of sound relate to setting intentions and the heart chakra? We can consider our intentions "words"—both spoken and unspoken. Our "gross" level of speaking our intentions can be considered to be at the vaikari, or most physical, level and reflect our expectations.

But through this Vedic framework, we can move even more deeply into consciousness and expand the power of our intentions. Through the heart chakra, which unites the physical and spiritual worlds, we expand our awareness and sense of self beyond our conditioning into deeper states of consciousness greater in both subtlety and connection with the wider expanse of consciousness available to us. This is where we can invite consciousness itself to cocreate with us, through us, and not just for us.

Anahata chakra, or the heart chakra, is where we move beyond the "me" consciousness into a wider, more connected "we" consciousness. This is depicted by the six-pointed star shown in the heart chakra, as shown in figure 13.2. The six-pointed star with one triangle pointing downward and one pointing upward reflects the promise of connecting the energies of the first, second, and third chakras upward into the heart, along with the energies of the spiritual planes from the crown, third eye, and throat chakras downward into the heart. When these energies meet in our heart, they help us bridge the physical and spiritual worlds and experience a higher level of consciousness in the anahata chakra. That is why the heart is also often described in many cultures, including the Vedic tradition, as the seat of the soul.

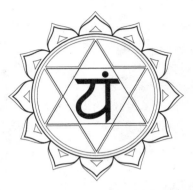

FIGURE 13.2. The *anahata*, or heart, chakra in Vedic tradition is considered a key chakra for spiritual assistance and serves as a gateway between the physical and spiritual worlds.

THE ANCIENT AND MODERN SCIENCE OF RITUAL

Although placebo research has shown that expectations are huge drivers of our self-healing effects down to the neural level, other placebo elements also show us the power of our behavior and minds to affect our healing. Another powerful element is ritual.

Ritual has been known in every culture to align the spirit-mind-body in ways that can augment the healing process by fostering a deepening of consciousness to bring about healing responses through specific intentions. Shamanistic cultures are perhaps the most discussed with respect to healing ritual—their rituals overtly call Spirit into the healing process.[12] An adept spiritual healer or shaman who follows a specific process dependent on intention and tradition generally uses dance, prayers, song, and specific elements of nature both to show reverence to Spirit in the healing process and to call for assistance. The shaman often describes leaving ordinary waking reality or entering a "trance state" to make contact with nature or other spirits to aid in the process of healing an individual or a tribe.[13] In many ways, this aspect of healing ritual (connection with and assistance from spirit guides) is echoed by modern-day biofield therapy practitioners, who often report calling in guides to work with them in the healing process.[14]

Ritual doesn't just occur between a shaman and a recipient of healing or a health-care practitioner and a patient. We engage in it daily—whether it's that first cup of coffee and reading the daily news or a shower before bed.

Rituals are a set of behaviors and an environment we use to cue our body-minds to a certain time of day (morning) or activity (time to sleep).

I am suggesting that you are already likely engaging in one or more rituals that affect your healing process, whether you are aware of it or not—and that by consciously creating a ritual meant for healing that engages your body, mind, and spirit, you allow your healing intention to fully manifest itself.

PUTTING IT INTO PRACTICE
Forming Your Healing Ritual

The most important part of ritual is consistency. The purpose of your creating and engaging in your own ritual is to train your body-mind to connect with your spirit to augment your healing process.

Opening to Your Healing Intention

Your ritual does not need to be overtly spiritual or complex. You get to decide what it looks like. Simple is beautiful here because you want something that's easy to do every day. Here are the first two steps:

1. **Create a sacred space.** This is a place you can physically go that is just for your healing ritual practice during the time that you practice. It can be in a corner of a room, or it can be somewhere outside. If the space has to be used for other purposes during the day, that's fine—but try to pick a quiet place at home where you can go when it's time to do your healing ritual. Keep it free of electronics and other distractions. Feel free to decorate this space in a way that engages your sense of beauty, creativity, and Spirit. You can create an altar with natural, religious, or spiritual elements as you see fit. You can put paintings or pictures around the area to remind you of inspiring beings or people you feel might aid you in your healing process. Or, you can keep it quiet,

simple, and uncluttered. Create a space that you feel best invites you to relax, be in the present moment, and open to Spirit.

2. **Create a sacred time.** I recommend engaging in your healing ritual in the morning, if possible (I know this is a lot to ask for most of us). If you can spare even five minutes for your ritual before fully engaging in your day, I highly recommend it. Before bed is another ideal time to engage in your healing ritual, when you can release the activities and thoughts of the day. Ideally, give yourself at least fifteen minutes for your healing ritual, and feel free to do it more than once a day, but you must commit to one consistent time of day you engage in your ritual.

After you've created your sacred space and identified your sacred time, you're ready to engage in your healing ritual. Here are some suggestions to create your ritual; please feel free to use these or create your own ritual steps as you see fit.

1. **Ground, connect, and fill up with energy.** Use the exercises in chapter 10 to bring yourself fully into your body. Feel the base of your spine and your feet, whether you choose to lie down, sit, or stand. Allow your body to rest in the position you've chosen and be fully open to receiving the energy of the Earth. Bring the energy of the Earth all the way up your body to the crown of your head. (If it feels more comfortable to bring energy from the crown of your head down your body, that's perfectly fine; just make sure you can feel your feet.)

2. **Create an invocation.** This is basically a chant, prayer, sound, or word that honors Spirit, in whatever form or fashion resonates the most deeply with you. If you connect with a specific religion, offer a chant, hymn, or prayer. If that isn't your preference, simply

create a sound or word that's comfortable, such as "ahhhhhhh," and opens up the heart and the solar plexus chakras. Creating sound through your body is a powerful way to ignite your attention and energy, thus helping to bring the mind and vital force together. When you first start doing this, say your invocation out loud, with sweetness and vigor combined. You can focus your attention on your heart chakra when you share your invocation. Over time, as your invocation begins to feel more and more powerful and present in your body, you might choose to say it silently and explore its effects. However, to achieve the power of unspoken sound, you must be comfortable with creating and feeling vibration—so I recommend starting with sound you can make out loud in the beginning. This will also help to open your throat chakra and release any fears you have about being heard.

3. **Give yourself the present of presence.** Now that you've created the energetic conditions to be connected, present, and ready to receive, allow yourself to do so. After sounding your invocation, simply enjoy the silence of the present moment by attending to your own breath, with nothing further to do for this brief time. Practice breathing in your body, using the Five-Breath Body Tune-In I shared with you in chapter 11 for at least five minutes, or more as you wish. You might feel different sensations in your body as you continue to breathe, and you'll likely be aware of thoughts. Allow the sensations and thoughts to come and go without clinging to any or dwelling on the meaning of this or that one. Simply return to and enjoy your breath in this moment, knowing there is nothing else you need to do at this time.

4. **Explore your healing intention.** After enjoying your breath and coming into presence, focus on your heart chakra. While holding awareness here, simply ask yourself the question: What wishes to

come into healing today? Allow yourself not to judge the answer, and don't worry if the answer doesn't become clear right away. You are simply creating the space for your unconscious desire to show itself. This is how you get a deeper clue to what your body and spirit want—which might or might not be what your conscious mind is saying. You might get an answer in a bodily sensation, image, sound, thought, or even a smell that connects with something meaningful for your healing process. If and when you get an answer, thank yourself and return back to your breath and your body. (If you don't get an answer, don't worry—just go on to the next step.)

5. **Cultivate your healing volition.** This is about strengthening your will and your energy for healing, whether for yourself or someone else. After you receive information on what is asking to be healed, begin to connect even more deeply with your body and breath. Focus specifically on your belly and solar plexus, the area between your belly button and heart. Bring to this area the golden light of the sun, and allow it to fill your insides through the belly. Initially, this might feel like an imagery exercise, but in time you will feel this viscerally in your body. You are nourishing your solar plexus, or manipura chakra, with the energy, or prana, required to carry out your healing desire. Feel this prana enter you from the middle of your body, from the front of your body, from the back of your body. Let this pure energy fill you inside so that you can feel both the top and bottom half of your body unite at your belly, bathed in brilliant yellow and orange light. Now, with this energy inside you, if a clear desire for healing came for you during this exercise, bring that desired healing effect (i.e., how you will feel after this healing takes place) to your mind, and then let it go. Let go of all details and planning, release your healing desire and intention from inside you, and simply feel the energy move within and through you.

6. **Close your ritual with gratitude.** Place your attention at your heart, and give thanks to any guides you feel aiding you in your healing process. Thank yourself for giving yourself the time for your healing ritual. Give thanks to the people and situations aiding you in your healing process. Close with a chant, prayer, or sound that resonates with you.

I recommend engaging in your healing ritual every day if you can. If that feels difficult for you at first, please try to do it three times a week and write about what you notice in the coming weeks as you make a healing ritual part of your life.

...

CHAPTER 14

Connect to Heal

As I write this chapter, hundreds of thousands of people around the world have died from Covid-19, and we are all grappling with reducing the spread of the virus. The pandemic has turned everything upside down, and although governments and global health groups are doing their best to control the situation, it's hard to predict what will happen next. The economy is shifting tremendously—nearly all people and businesses have been financially affected. Understandably, the natural human response has people moving somewhere along the emotional spectrum from denial to panic to shock. Yet many doctors and public health experts have been predicting this type of pandemic for years and warn of more to come.[1] It wasn't a question of "if" but "when"—and for how long? Sheltering in place might become a regular habit.

All of us sheltering in place are learning deep lessons about the importance and meaning of human connection. How do we reconcile the mandates of social distancing with the fact that we are biologically wired to connect?

We've likely heard the phrase "loneliness kills," and many of us are familiar with the neuroscience, public health studies, and social science that not only acknowledge this but also show the pathways by which loneliness kills.[2] Just to give you an idea, poor social connection is a greater predictor of premature death than tobacco use, obesity, and excessive alcohol use.[3]

The flip side of the science of loneliness is that connection heals—an even stronger truth. As human beings, we are social creatures—we thrive on connection down to our cells. Social connection has been studied in depth for decades by scientists in neuroscience, psychology, psychoneuroimmunology (PNI), psychoneuroendocrinology (PNE), and public health. We study social connection in terms of quantity and type (e.g., social integration, social isolation, and social networks) and perceived quality (e.g., closeness, loneliness, and social support).

The combined results of these studies so strongly support the vital impact of social connection on our health that many scientists have called for governments to advance social connection as a public health priority.

How strong are the effects of improving social connection on our health? Here are some highlights:

A meta-analysis combined data over 148 studies to find that being more socially connected is related to a 50 percent reduced risk of early death.[4]

Higher levels of social support are associated with less cardiovascular disease, including atherosclerosis.

Higher social support is related to lower blood pressure as well as less cardiovascular reactivity to stress.[5]

Higher levels of social support are related to decreased inflammation in women and men.[6]

Many of us might be familiar with the results of these studies. But we might not have appreciated just how dynamic the effects of connection are. Regardless of our previous or current social status, our trauma histories, or our health histories, each of us has immense power to jump-start ours and others' healing process by doing a simple thing: fostering positive social connections in whatever form is available to us. Connection isn't just a numbers game. The data suggest that quality, not simply quantity, of our social relationships matters, especially as we get older. One study from researchers at the University of Rochester followed hundreds of people over a period of thirty years to observe whether social quality or quantity predicted better psychological outcomes, including less depression and increased well-being, at age fifty. The data revealed that for increased psychological well-being, quantity seemed to matter more for people in their twenties, whereas quality seemed to matter more for people in their thirties.[7] The authors proposed that a wider social network might help foster opportunities for social mobility and connection in younger life, whereas cultivating close relationships with a trusted network is more beneficial in later life. Because we are connected, we can feel each others' joy and each others' pain—down to our neurons.

Groundbreaking controlled experiments with neuroimaging (specifically, functional magnetic resonance imaging, or fMRI) by Naomi Eisenberger and colleagues at the University of California–Los Angeles demonstrated how social rejection lights up the same brain pathways as physical pain—and that these pathways light up in our brains even when we witness the pain of another.[8]

HEALING CONNECTION: THE SPIRITUAL AND BIOENERGETIC PERSPECTIVE

Human beings are by nature creative creatures. When one avenue closes to us to connect, such as spending time one-on-one in person, we find other pathways to connect. Even in our screen-overload culture, we've figured out how our current technologies can be used for connection and social good. At this point during the Covid-19 crisis, we can still connect through the internet, using Zoom to have virtual dinners with family and friends, satsangs, and other spiritual gatherings. Even a good, old-fashioned phone conversation with a dear friend has reemerged as a deeper way to connect. All of these methods of communication through technology are meaningful for maintaining our health and are likely influencing our physiology, whether we connect in person or by video chats.

But most of us are not as aware of our innate "technologies" for connection, such as sending lovingkindness to someone, whether near or far. Research by Kathi Kemper at the University of Ohio has demonstrated that a person can send someone else lovingkindness (whether the recipient knows loving-kindness is being sent or not), and this can decrease the recipient's stress and increase his or her heart rate variability and sense of peace.[9] Kemper's results suggest that we can feel lovingkindness fairly immediately even when we don't know someone is sending it to us. This further empowers us to know that sending compassion and love to another might have a meaningful effect for another's healing—whether they know you are sending them love or not.

Practices such as lovingkindness meditation are rooted in an understanding that our fundamental interconnection has nothing to do with physical proximity to each other. Experienced meditators from many different traditions, for example, speak of a practice-based understanding of the interconnectedness of all life based on a felt experience of interrelationship, or "inter-being," as described by Buddhist teacher Thich Nhat Hanh.[10] The experience of the "self" expands to understand that "you" and "I" are not separate but, in fact, part of an interconnected whole. Practiced meditators from contemplative traditions across the world often experience the "self" dissolve into pure nothingness, sometimes also called the "void" or "emptiness" in several Buddhist traditions.[11] Our experience of the self beyond the physical being, even beyond time and space, is therefore not limited by our physical-mental condition.[12] Similar experiences of "ego dissolution" are also described in entheogen (psychedelic) research, in which entheogen-guided journeys with a trained professional can help a person's sense of self expand beyond egoic, conditioned consciousness, providing for greater insight and perspective into the human condition, the nature of interconnection, and insights for personal healing, including from trauma.[13]

Of course, when we think of connection, we think of the heart. In many traditions the heart chakra plays an important role in healing connections. Anahata chakra, the heart chakra, as we discussed in chapter 13, helps us connect to and process deep emotions such as love and grief (see figure 14.1). Opening our hearts can also help us viscerally connect with other people's feelings. The heart chakra is also a gateway for connection with Spirit, and the connection with Spirit aids us in amplifying love and healing for each other. Put simply, by focusing on the heart and deepening our abilities to feel others as well as ourselves, we open to even deeper levels of being and allow for deeper levels of connective healing.

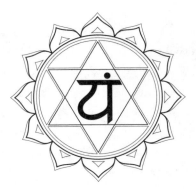

FIGURE 14.1. The fourth chakra, called *anahata* chakra in Tantric and Vedic traditions. Anahata, or "unstruck sound," refers to the different levels of consciousness that can be accessed through this chakra. In Vedic and Tantric traditions, this chakra is generally associated with the element of air.

PUTTING IT INTO PRACTICE
Cultivating Strong Social Connections for Healing

We can learn from scientific research on connection, spiritual traditions, and health crises such as Covid-19 that connection is vital for our health and the health of the planet. We also know there are many ways we can connect—whether emotionally, energetically, mentally, physically, sexually, or spiritually (and sometimes, all of these at once!). The key for us is to have tools at hand to foster connections to heal ourselves and others when we need them most and not feel powerless to connect if we can't do so by our preferred means. Here are some common-sense tips for making the most of your biological and spiritual wiring for connection, whether in person or otherwise:

1. **Listen deeply, with your heart as well as your ears.** Deep listening is a skill and requires stillness. When we have tons going on in our minds, we feel the need to unload, and others do as well. Have you ever noticed how it feels to be in or witness a "parallel conversation," where neither person is really listening to the other but simply unloading his or her thoughts and emotions in sequence? It might feel cathartic, but the healing relationship can only go so far.

Deep listening is an art and requires us to be still as well as present in our bodies. When we engage in deep listening, we not only listen to the words but also we are sensitive to tone of voice as well as body posture and energy, which tell us a person's true emotional state when they are speaking. Sometimes we just need to bear witness. Listening is healing in and of itself. Listening allows us to be really present with each other, even if it means listening to problems without feeling the need to give advice or fix people or their issues.

2. **Be a mentor or mentee.** We are all surrounded by ordinary heroes and heroines who might not have millions of Facebook followers but in whom we can take refuge, whose presence itself is healing, and from whom we think we can learn something. Although we are all busy, if you are blessed to be people's ordinary hero/heroine, try to make some time for them when they ask for it. Likewise, don't be too shy to ask for occasional time with someone or reach out for advice or help from someone you respect and trust when you need it. Whatever amount of time you can commit to being a mentor or mentee, whether virtually or in person, it can make a world of difference for you and others. This will open your heart to experience one of love's greatest reflections—service.

3. **Take time to foster and heal family relationships.** Mother Teresa famously said, "If you want to change the world, go home and love your family." It's such a wise saying, given the sacred wounds of family life combined with the busy-ness of day-to-day life. We might think our purpose is "out there," doing something important for the world, and forget that the whole point of life is to be in a state of love. Who better to be in love with than your family?

    We might not feel particularly wounded by family dynamics (although I've yet to meet anyone who said he or she came from a perfect family)—but the general truth is, our ways of interacting with others come straight out of the family dynamics in which we were raised. When we are able to spend time with family members and talk about unhealthy dynamics in a peaceful fashion without blame, guilt, or shame (e.g., "when this happens . . . I feel . . . and I wish we could. . ."), spontaneous healing takes place.

For some of us, the idea of going back to our family of origin to help heal sacred wounds might feel impossible or even inadvisable. In those cases, we can simply rest our awareness on how we are responding to our current situation and the people around us. Do we have blind spots in friendships, romantic relationships, or work relationships that tend to end badly, but we don't know why? Do we avoid close relationships with others, and if so, is there something about our childhood dynamics that might relate to that? We can work with a good therapist to uncover and help untangle ourselves from a history of unhealthy family dynamics that hang up our abilities to have joyful relationships. We can also work on clearing away patterns of unhealthy dynamics on the bioenergetic or spiritual level (see the exercise below).

4. **Do fun things with those you love.** Sadly, sometimes the ones we love the most don't get the best of us. Life gets in the way. We are too busy cooking, cleaning, meeting deadlines, organizing, taking care of children, working, or doing other essential life tasks to realize we might not be making enough time to enjoy the people we love the most. Working parents of young children know this well—they are often adult-time deprived, food deprived, and sleep deprived. If they have a moment at all to themselves (possibly in the bathroom), it's just enough to breathe until it's full on to the next task. For others who don't have children or whose children are grown, it's still easy to get so incredibly busy that we forget to make time for others.

However, the best thing we can do for our sanity and our relationships is to take even fifteen minutes of uninterrupted "fun time" with a loved one every day—whether it's a child, friend, pet, or spouse. This is simply unstructured time in which there is absolutely no goal except to enjoy each other's company. You can, for example, play a spontaneous game or dance with your children and simply follow their lead. You can ask a partner or friend to go hang out in the park with you and simply let spontaneity lead your next steps. You can take a wandering walk with a pet on which there is no particular destination or any agenda to discuss anything or get anything done. Allowing for sacred, spontaneous time with family and friends allows for creativity and fun to guide your time together and opens up new possibilities for experience in your relationships.

ADVANCED PRACTICE: HEALING OUR RELATIONSHIPS

Those of us who feel called to work with the biofield to heal particular relationships can engage in simple practices that help us recognize and release unwanted relational patterns on the subtle energetic level. We can also work with the biofield to foster healing for others on the spiritual level. Feel free to use these basic practices in the following exercise and integrate them into your healing rituals as you see fit.

Healing Relationships: A Biofield Exercise

1. Follow steps 1–3 of Opening to Your Healing Intention in chapter 13 (in other words, first start by grounding, sounding an invocation, and becoming present in your body).

2. Now, instead of exploring your intention (step 4 in that ritual), set a specific intention to heal a relationship between yourself and someone else. Take a few moments to do this, and allow any images and sensations to come to mind while staying grounded and breathing deeply into your body.

3. If the intention is specifically to release/separate yourself from a person to gain healthier relationship dynamics or space, grow your healing volition by staying grounded and cultivating a strong light source in your body. Feel your feet firmly planted on the Earth, and feel the Earth's energy rising from the ground up your legs to your navel. Now bring the light of the sun (you can visualize this to make it easier) into your navel, and let it grow so that your entire body feels strong with this inner light of pure energy and strength. Let it fill your heart and your entire being. Make sure you are feeling grounded (connected with the Earth) throughout the process and releasing any discomfort or pain down your legs into the Earth. Now bring to mind the other person, and let your mind's eye notice how this person's energy form does or does not come into your field. If you notice tendrils, tubes, or cords connecting this person to you, and you do not wish to have them there, you will "cut the cord" by simply applying light, like a laser, to it. As you cut the cord, state an affirmation that feels right to you, such as, "By cutting this cord I release all unhealthy dynamics between us and reclaim my whole self energetically." Continue applying light to any cords until you feel the process is complete and your energy feels stable and strong. Notice the energetic changes in your body.

    If needed, you can ask this person to stay distant from you by simply asking them to return to their light source and energetically "pushing" them away from your field—if needed, as far as outer space! After this is complete, wish for this person their best and highest good while affirming your sovereignty and space. This practice is best done when we are not in a state of anger but in a state of peaceful resolve and strength.

4. If the intention is simply to foster greater healing and harmony with another person, while staying grounded, bring your awareness to your heart chakra, in the middle of your chest. Allow any feelings, whether emotional or kinesthetic, you feel in your heart to simply be there, and be with the emotions or sensations. After you feel somewhat settled, ask any inner guidance (whether your inner self, soul, higher Consciousness, Spirit, or guides) to be with you in your heart chakra. Allow yourself to lean back ever so slightly to feel guidance come energetically from the back of your heart center, as if you can feel your inner guidance enveloping you in a hug. Allow yourself to feel that strength and support. From this place, tune in to the other person (it does not matter if he or she is near or far from you) by imagining that you can see this person in front of you. See what your intuition tells you about this person's state, and just notice what you get.

    Now bring into your heart chakra a sincere wish for the greatest level of well-being for this person. Visualize that if it helps, but really feel yourself connect in the form of light and loving feelings to this person for just a few minutes (even two to three minutes can be sufficient). You may use the phrases often used in lovingkindness meditation, which include: "May you be safe. May you be happy. May you be free from suffering. May you be at peace." After sending this energy of love and sincere wishes for well-being, release yourself energetically from this person, and thank your Guidance for helping you with this process. Notice that in this exercise, you are not specifically trying to create energetic cords of relationship with that person but simply wishing him or her well. Simply by wishing the other person well and cultivating a field of emotional, mental, and spiritual positivity around him or her, you will notice shifts in your relationship dynamics. In this process, we begin to use the heart and connection to Guidance to help us better heal ourselves and others.

. . .

As you practice these exercises, feel free to use my audio meditation "The Heart's Guidance" at shaminijain.com/bookresources to touch into your heart on these energetic and spiritual levels to foster deeper connection with yourself and your inner guidance and strengthen your heart and lungs in the process.

Now that we've learned about the power of connection and have been fostering a deeper sense of connection between ourselves and our inner guidance, let's explore the power of spiritual connection even more deeply in chapter 15, on surrender.

CHAPTER 15

Surrender

Not too long ago, I had the privilege of meeting with and having healing sessions with a South American healer, whom I will call Clara. A colleague had invited me to meet Clara and experience her healing because he believed she was on the level of a "saint." She did not advertise herself in any way, however, because she didn't want to be in the spotlight as a healer. Much like my first-ever healing session in Santa Cruz, I was happy to have a session and simply curious to see what would happen. Clara asked me if I had any physical ailments. Interestingly, at the moment none came to mind—despite the fact that I actually had been suffering for a few years with what appeared to be perimenopausal symptoms. The symptoms seemed to be wreaking havoc on my sleep and immunity in particular. I just chalked it up to hormone changes and my choice to live a constantly on-the-go lifestyle as a middle-aged woman. Although I gave Clara no indication that I had anything physically wrong with me, she told me right away I had a complication. "What I see is a liquid tumor behind your thyroid that is causing problems with your hormones. It is complex and significant. If . . ." she hesitated. "If I was not to try to fix this at this time, it would calcify and could become a cancer."

"Oh." Well, that statement floored me, as you might imagine. I had been feeling heat and some level of discomfort in my throat for several months but chalked it up to an energetic imbalance because of overdoing it with all the singing performances. Having been in the heavy metal tribute band for a few years, I had begun to notice feeling fatigued after our rehearsals and shows.

"I currently sing in a heavy metal tribute band. Could my singing this music regularly be part of the reason this 'liquid tumor' has formed?"

After Clara laughed and, like most, admitted she really didn't see me as a heavy metal singer, she took a moment to check in with her guidance, then said point blank, "Yes. You will have to phase it out, and maybe eventually stop altogether. It is not that you have to stop singing entirely—that would be like telling a bird it could not fly—singing is part of your nature. But this forceful singing that you are doing . . ." she paused. "You are straining yourself to sing in this way, and that is the problem. You will have to stop it. . . . In general, you are not allowing Spirit to come into your body fully, so you are not receiving its full Wisdom."

"Oh." I paused. "Well, I have a big gig coming up in a few weeks . . . are you saying I should cancel it?"

At this point Clara looked at me in amazement and shock. Clearly I was not listening. "Tu no entiendes!" she exclaimed. "Si no para, *cancer*!" ("You don't understand! If you don't stop, *cancer*!")

I did not want to hear this. I was not willing to give up singing, again, after having stopped for so many years. I loved the band, the creative expression, the full-force singing, and the love from our fans. Now I was being told I had to give it all up, again. I burst into tears like a child because my inner child's dreams of being a rock star were coming to an end.

Clearly, there was a deep spiritual lesson here.

The session with Clara was completely life-changing for me. I couldn't confirm or deny what she had said about the liquid tumor because I didn't go to a doctor to get a blood test before or after I saw her. After my healing sessions with her, I did notice an immediate difference in my bodily energy as well as in my throat. The burning in my throat had gone away, and my energy felt more even, with fewer bursts of strong energy coupled with exhaustion. But the most profound effect I noticed was how I felt emotionally and spiritually. I had a sense of deep peace, contentment, and connection to what

I call Spirit—a higher guidance I could feel surrounding me with a sense of ease, grace, and spiritual love I felt for weeks, if not months, afterward.

I also began to understand that the heavy metal singing was a reflection of how I was choosing to live my life—driven by force and not respecting my body or my spirit. I wasn't just pushing my voice, I was pushing my life—to the point of gross imbalance. I believed in the mission of my nonprofit, Consciousness and Healing Initiative (CHI), and having sacrificed significant effort, money, and time for several years, I was determined to make it work. As a result, I took every speaking and teaching engagement I could get, if it paid enough to help sustain my family. At home, I pushed to be a supermom as best I could—I was hands-on with my family, making sure that I spent quality time with the kids, that everyone was fed appropriately, that the dishes were done, and that everything was in order. I said yes to every singing gig because I needed a way to get out of my head and be in creative flow and have fun. I was largely ignoring my husband's clear unhappiness with the frenetic patterns of life I set up for us. I wanted it all, I wanted it now, and I wasn't willing to give up anything.

This healing session, I realized, was not just about too much heavy metal singing. It was a wake-up call about the perils of living a forced, unbalanced life full of ego-driven ambition, albeit with good intentions for serving others.

SURRENDER: A SPIRITUAL PERSPECTIVE

Opportunities for spiritual surrender often occur to remind us that coming into our sheer Being is all that is actually required for spiritual growth, and when we forget this, our circumstances shift to help us remember. When we wholly align with our unique life purpose, or dharma, we do not need to try. We are simply in nonegoic flow, the opposite of egoic force. I had experienced this dharmic flow, which led me to start the nonprofit with my colleagues. But as I fell into my fears about financial sustainability, I created anxiety patterns for myself that made me feel I needed to work harder and push in every direction. Not in spite of but because of my best efforts, I was paradoxically blocking my flow and my desire to serve by valuing myself as a human *doing* through egoic will, not a human *being* in trusted relationship with myself, my loved ones, and Spirit.

Blessings that require surrender can sometimes appear mixed and can even provoke anxiety because they often require us to let go of our attachments in order to fully receive and trust what is to come next. This process of surrender is not easy. It requires us to become grounded in the present. It calls for a curiosity for what lies ahead and a fully open heart to receive it as well as release what no longer serves our path. It requires strong trust in our inner guidance and the wisdom to discern what Spirit tells us versus what others say. We have to find and feel our deepest desires and then release them. We have to find our deepest fears, look them in the eye, and release those as well. In the process of recognizing and releasing these attachments (whether desires, fears, or both), we become more present with our true selves and more fully able to receive, live joyfully, and serve others.

As we continue to live a path of purpose and service, we realize our life is not fully our own—that is, our life is not only for our egoic fulfillment. We recognize that expanding our consciousness and our relationships with others are one and the same, and that sacrifice is, in fact, related to expansion in consciousness and relationships. As our hearts open more fully, so does our recognition of interdependence. We realize that "our" lives are really a web of shared lives, and "personal sacrifices" are actually wise decisions made for the good of the whole that also refine and reflect our true being.

The global Covid-19 crisis is a perfect example of how, if practiced wisely, the natural processes of sacrifice and surrender can help heal and foster a flourishing society and a sustainable Earth. As we deepen our relationships with all beings, we can recognize and feel our interdependence. Compassion and love naturally spring forth from those actions and feelings. As we see our interconnections, whether with family members, perfect strangers in our town, or ants—not only do we wish not to harm those beings but also we wish to take care of them because we realize they are not separate from us. When we create divisions between us as living beings, we suffer because we don't recognize the fundamental truth that healing our suffering and healing someone else's suffering is reciprocal. We are all part of a unified wholeness and, therefore, connected.

When we release our attachment to something for the greater good—such as relinquishing meat to prevent harm to animals or avoiding nondegradable plastic products to prevent harm to the Earth—it often might not feel like a sacrifice because we are so rooted in our love of animals and the Earth. But when the sacrifice appears to counter our everyday happiness, we often question it.

I recognize that what I am saying might be triggering for some of you, particularly those of you who might have experienced manipulation or abuse in relationships. "Sacrifice" and "surrender" often feel like dirty words to many of us, especially women. We might relate them with being brainwashed or having a martyr complex.

In fact, surrender is not a true loss of control—it's a loss of false control. Surrender is allowing your spirit instead of your conditioned mind to guide your life. The true practice of surrender is a spiritual growth process that allows you to live your life more deeply as who you truly are. Surrender requires trust in your innermost being and in a higher power. Sacrifice is, essentially, an act that reflects surrender—it allows you to release what no longer serves you. It is relinquishment of an ego attachment in order to grow your spiritual self. In my view, sacrifice is not necessarily needed for surrender, but when we are attached to something that impedes our spiritual evolution, we need to relinquish that attachment.

THE SCIENCE AND SPIRITUALITY OF SURRENDER

In my view, there is a serious dearth of research on cultural descriptions, health impacts, and processes of surrender. In the West, the concept has mostly been discussed in the context of alcoholism and spirituality, most specifically within the twelve-step program and in Christian traditions.[1] Spiritual surrender is beginning to be researched more seriously by psychologists. Some studies indicate that those who engage in spiritual surrender tend to have reduced anxiety and stress.[2]

Interestingly, the first few steps in the twelve-step program steer the person struggling with addiction to surrender to a higher power because its leaders believe the participants must acknowledge their limitations in being able to fight the demon of addiction—without spiritual help (some would even say Divine guidance and support, or God's support). This might seem like a cop-out to some (shouldn't we be able to handle our own problems instead of saying "I can't do it" and passing it off to God?).

However, this first step of surrendering to a higher power can also be viewed as an acknowledgment of the limitations of our conditioning. We are human beings, born and raised in certain environments, exposed to both happy and traumatic events, and shaped by our culture—some to a greater degree than others. This is all reflected in our conditioned self. For those who experienced a significant amount of conflict or trauma without good modeling of how to handle it, addiction emerges from struggles to try to cope with negative emotional states such as stress and trauma. Our conditioning can lead us down a path of destruction, and we need to explore beyond our conditioned self to get the answer. As Albert Einstein said, you can't solve a problem with the same kind of thinking that created the problem! When we identify with the conditioned self only, we are incomplete because our conditioned experience itself is incomplete. If we identify only with the conditioned self—that is, our families of origin, our habits, our past experiences—we trap ourselves into a smaller and sometimes more circular life in which we keep repeating past mistakes in a pattern we can't seem to stop.

To surrender when struggling with any addiction (and we are all addicted to something) means acknowledging the pattern that must be interrupted and understanding that our conditioned mind cannot show ourselves the solution on its own. When we surrender, we recognize that a wider perspective exists—and that by opening to that perspective and more possibilities, we can foster our hopes and dreams into reality instead of living our conditioned nightmares. But we must open to that realm by acknowledging that we need help—we need input from a reality bigger than our small, conditioned selves.

The understandings of surrender in these psychotherapeutic and religious traditions are similar to those in Eastern philosophy—the process of surrender acknowledges our human imperfections and asks us to connect with our understanding of the highest power to help guide and shape our life toward one of peace and union with the Divine—and often to better lead a life of service.[3] Although the process of devotion in traditions such as *bhakti* yoga is not often described as surrender, a bhakti yogi will tell you that the process is absolutely a surrender to the Divine. Devotional practices transform egoic desires into an earnest seeking of Divine union—resulting in significant experiences of Grace and growth.

THE ENERGY OF SURRENDER:
THE CHAKRA PERSPECTIVE

Two chakras merit specific mention in terms of how they relate to surrender: the anahata, or heart, chakra (see figure 15.1), and the *sahasrara*, or crown, chakra (see figure 15.2). When we focus on our heart, we are sending a signal to ourselves to move from the thinking, conditioned mind into feeling and connection. If we intend to foster a deeper connection with divine guidance, the heart chakra's energy will help foster that.

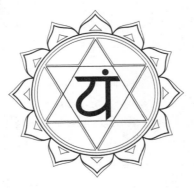

FIGURE 15.1 The fourth chakra, called *anahata* chakra in Tantric and Vedic traditions, is generally associated with the element of air. In many traditions, the heart chakra is considered a gateway to feel devotion and open to divine Grace.

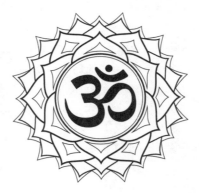

FIGURE 15.2. The *sahasrara*, or crown, chakra in Vedic and Tantric traditions allows us to fully realize and connect with the Divine.

The sahasrara chakra, or crown chakra, is above the top of the head. *Sahasrara* can be translated as "thousand-petaled," and this chakra is depicted by a thousand-petaled white lotus. This chakra is sometimes also called *brahmarandhra*, or doorway to God.[4]

The crown chakra is a portal to what has been described as the experience of God, nonduality, Oneness, and pure Consciousness beyond space and time. This can be transient or permanent. For example, Buddhist, Jain, Tantric, and Vedic lineages have described how a fully opened crown chakra helps us to realize our divine nature as being One with Consciousness—as we explored in chapter 3, these are often described as particular types of *samadhi* states often not permanent in nature.[5] Those qualities of Consciousness, as you might remember, are reflected by the words *sat-chit-ananda* ("truth," "Consciousness," and "bliss"). The crown chakra and the experience of sat-chit-ananda ("all knowing," "true," and "ever blissful") that can be gained through it reminds us that in addition to helping us fight our own demons, the process of surrender leads to true enjoyment because now we can fully realize ourselves as cocreators, with Spiritual guidance, to foster a bigger dream beyond our egoic desires. As our consciousness expands, we recognize that our deepest desires—to be whole, to be free, to live with ease and joy—are shared with all creatures, and we can abide in bliss by intellectually understanding and actually experiencing these deeper truths of expansion. Uniting the heart and crown chakras plays a key role in surrender because it allows us to carry our devotion for the Divine to be in direct contact and communion with the Divine. This is where we are given spiritual wisdom and guidance to live our lives in accordance with divine principles—in other words, to live beyond a life that can be tortured by circular, egoic conditioning, including addictions.

PUTTING IT INTO PRACTICE
Exploring Sacrifice and Surrender

For a guided, chakra-based meditation that uses the gift of every chakra for releasing what we don't need and helps us connect more deeply with the Divine, you can listen to my "Embodied Surrender" meditation, available at shaminijain.com/bookresources. However, please remember that the chakras are just one way of pointing a pathway toward surrender and union with the Divine. Use the spiritual practices, names, and devotional processes that resonate with you most deeply to connect with your Divine Source.

CONSIDERING THE NEED FOR A SACRIFICE

As we discussed above, considering a sacrifice or "letting go" might be useful if you find you're attached to something or someone not serving your healing process or your life. However, if you have a history of being abused, bullied, or manipulated—the idea of sacrifice, especially if suggested by another person, can feel scary. Given that, it's important to ask yourself the following questions when you consider the need to sacrifice something:

What is the habit/person/situation/thing of which I am being asked to let go?

What is the meaning of that habit/person/situation/thing to me? What happens if I let it go? What am I afraid of losing (or gaining) as a result?

Is this habit/person/situation/thing serving my highest good? Does it align with my values and purpose?

Who is asking me to let go of this, and why? (If it's another person, and the sacrifice being asked of you does not serve your highest good, reconsider. Ultimately, true sacrifice is born out of a willingness to surrender—for your soul's evolution, not for someone else's satisfaction.)

Am I willing to let go of this habit/person/situation/thing and see what happens next, even if I don't know what it is? If so, are there situations or people that can support me during this transition?

If you ask these questions and open your heart to receive the answers, you'll know whether the sacrifice being asked of you is part of your spiritual growth process and whether you're ready to trust and take the leap to surrender to it.

FOSTERING THE PROCESS OF SURRENDER

How do you know if engaging in a process of surrender is right for you?

You feel stuck, like you've been pushing or waiting for something, and it's not happening.

You feel like you're not in alignment with your values or heart's desires.

You feel angry, empty, or sad much of the time.

You feel out of control.

Others are concerned for your safety or health.

If you feel any of these things (and most of us do from time to time), then a simple surrender process will help you to realign with the flow of Divinity and bring you the true power you need to cocreate your next steps in life.

You will likely find your own process for opening to surrender, and if you follow a particular religious or spiritual practice, you might already be familiar with steps to surrender to the Divine. However, if you're just getting started or want to try something different, you can use the suggestions below. This is a practice you can integrate with your Opening to Your Healing Intention ritual from chapter 13.

Opening to Surrender

Here are guidelines for opening to surrender:

1. Connect with your sacred space. Use the same space you are using for your ritual (see chapter 13).

2. Begin your intention ritual. That is, follow steps 1–3 of the Opening to Your Healing Intention ritual at the end of chapter 13, with a few minutes of time devoted to each step. To remind you, these steps are:
    a. Ground—get into your body and connected with the Earth.
    b. Sound your invocation—prepare your body for Divine connection with a prayer, mantra, or sound as you see fit.
    c. Connect with Presence—allow yourself to feel your breath and your presence.

3. Invite Divine Presence to be with you. This is an intentional invitation to open to the wisdom and presence of that which you consider the ultimate source and substance of the Divine. You might call this Gaia, God, Soul, Spirit, or many other names. Simply ask silently that you be connected with this Divinity and that this Divinity guide you. You can focus your attention on your heart and the crown of your head when opening to the Divine.

4. Give reverence. Reverence can be considered the highest form of praise. It is a process of humbling our own egos and acknowledging that our conditioned selves can take us only so far. Reverence can be given with a devotional song, prayer, or simple words of reverence to the Divine—and can be shared silently as well as out loud, depending on what feels right to you.

5. Sit in silence with Divinity. In this space and time there is absolutely nothing to do but enjoy being in the presence of and connection with the Divine. If your mind needs something to focus on, I recommend that you focus on the crown of your head to allow for greater ease in connection and communication with the Divine. Allow any sensations or thoughts to simply pass through you, and do your best not to react to them.

6. Ask for guidance and strength. Once you feel the comfort, love, and nurturance of Divine presence and have allowed yourself to simply enjoy that presence, if you are struggling with a particular issue, simply ask for guidance and release the issue. If you need help releasing an addiction or attachment, ask for strength to help release this attachment from your life. If you are feeling stuck and need energy or direction to help you with next steps, ask the Divine to cocreate with you. Then hold silence so that this guidance can come through you. It might come in a burst of energy, images, words, or some other form and might come through during this time or later during the day.

7. Close with gratitude. Once you are ready to formally end your practice, close with reverence and gratitude for Divine Presence. Know that this presence is always with you, and thank yourself for giving yourself the time to explicitly connect.

...

The process of surrender is a lifelong process that ultimately leads us to experience Consciousness in its full form—so we can know our true nature—ever blissful, ever knowing, and ever present. Enjoy this process and the fruits of spiritual surrender because they bring you closest to the Source of Healing—your Divine Light.

AFTERWORD

Healing Futures

We are at a pivotal point in humanity's evolution. Our current climate crises, health crises, and social inequities reflect a great need for humanity to transform our way of acting, being, and thinking about the world. If we don't, we face real possibilities of greater suffering—even extinction. As heavy as that is, we have to look at the realities of where we are and what has gotten us here.

Given where we are in human history, we might take in all that we've just learned about biofield science and practice and still wonder: What is the real relevance of the biofield today, given the state of our world? The data, science, and thinking about the biofield are certainly groundbreaking. Yet these are more than just fascinating studies to talk about at a dinner party. These data are begging us to awaken to our human healing power and shift the way we experience each other and the world as a result.

When we look at all the data behind biofield healing, alongside the ancient wisdom that explained the practices, purposes, and spiritual cores from which these healing methods came, it reminds us of two fundamental truths crucial to remember and act on in our lives. One, we are fundamentally interconnected—down to our consciousness affecting another's healing. Two, we are far more powerful as agents of healing than we can ever imagine.

The biofield, and the science behind it, beseeches us to come to a full realization that we don't end here—we don't end at our skin. We are interconnected beings, both within and between our body-minds. The field of psychoneuroimmunology (PNI) has now shown us that separatist thinking, which made us think of our bodies as machines with different unrelated parts, is completely inaccurate. PNI and its related fields show just how powerful the mind-body is as a system—and, as a result, how powerful our emotional, mental, social, and spiritual states are for our health.

Where we were taught that a placebo is not real or involves trickery because it isn't a chemically active substance, we've realized that placebo research is actually telling us about the power of our emotions and minds to heal ourselves. And as we explore the biofield through the study of healing, we are further realizing how false and dated this idea of our separateness from our environment is. We realize how buying into this fallacy of separateness is greatly hurting us. When we believe in our separateness, when we don't see ourselves connected with each other and the Earth, we feel we are alone in our suffering and that nothing and nobody can really help us—that our suffering is simply because of bad genes, bad environments, or other factors beyond our control that can never be changed. We might feel that the only action we can take is to mask our symptoms with material things or substances and that we have no power over our own health. In the illusion of separateness, we also numb ourselves to each other's suffering instead of realizing we have the power to instantaneously alleviate someone else's pain—and even prevent that pain from occurring.

The biofield healing data are telling us that it is possible for a human being to send healing to others and not only reduce their suffering but also affect their health all the way to their physical bodies. The data already show that a person can send healing energy to an animal with cancer and affect its tumor down to the functions of cell signaling pathways and immune transmitters. Reports from patients suggest that a healer thousands of miles away can help foster healing of another's suffering—sometimes with life-changing results. How incredibly powerful and connected we are! How vast is our potential as human healing agents!

Biofield science and healing remind us that the key to our thriving as human beings is first simply to understand and believe in our power to realign our world into one commensurate with our highest human potential and not settle for the outdated thinking and, quite frankly, disempowering rhetoric that keeps us feeling divided and helpless.

What, specifically, will we do now to help scale up the future of biofield healing itself as a group of caring and committed citizens? **Believing** in healing possibilities is one step, and **actualizing**, making those possibilities a reality, is another. At our nonprofit, the Consciousness and Healing Initiative (CHI), we've considered this question quite a bit. Recently, we engaged in collaborative inquiry and planning to foster systems change for biofield healing.

Through interviews with more than sixty stakeholders in education, healing practice, policy, research, and technology, as well as a significant amount of expert analysis, we've created and shared a state-of-the-art report that summarizes what we know about the promise of biofield healing—and articulates key ongoing steps needed for healing systems change. Key steps include deepening our scientific inquiry through collaborative, interdisciplinary biofield science research at top-tier universities; communicating results of studies to the public as well as stakeholders in policy and health care; and developing biofield-based technology for preventative medicine diagnoses and treatment. Another key step includes providing evidence-based education on biofield-based self-care—that is, educating everyone on how to sense and work with their biofields to enhance their health and prevent disease. Our goal is to bring evidence-based healing into clinics and hospitals and foster self-care for all people. The report, systems change map, action plan, and more are freely available at our nonprofit's website, chi.is.

Our next immediate steps in scaling up healing include sharing perspectives of both scientists and healers with the broader global community. In general, healers need to have a greater voice at the table as we advance biofield research and technology as well as, of course, education and practice. This includes fully incorporating indigenous perspectives and indigenous wisdom holders in healing and medicine. Indigenous healing systems have always taught principles of holism and expressed that these principles are crucial to adopt for the healing of ourselves, each other, and the planet.

Understanding the fundamental interconnection between our bodies, climate change, our minds, our spirits, and the biofield as a connecting medium for healing is an example of indigenous wisdom ignored because of the colonization of medicine across the globe. In many ways, we need to go back to the future to mend the fractures in understanding that have kept us from believing that we have the power to heal ourselves and each other. It is time for us to listen deeply to the wisdom of the elders, who understand on a deep, embodied level how we can shift our entire way of being to one of harmony and interconnectedness instead of the fallacy of separateness, which causes more misery.

Perhaps most importantly, as the Jain nun told me at the beginning of my journey, healing starts first with each of us. In order for us to truly understand the mysteries and realities of healing, we must embark on the healing journey ourselves. For myself, I now believe that the path of healing and the path of spiritual liberation are one and the same. Healing isn't about just bringing us comfort, making a wound close faster, or taking away our pain (all of which might happen). Healing is fundamentally about realigning with our soul's force and power so that we live a life of harmony within ourselves, with each other, and with the planet. Through the path of healing, we learn to stop identifying with things not truly connected with our spirit, we can delight in the interconnections of our own being and being with others, and we can spread joy as well as feel others' pain. We can marvel at how nature heals herself and explore how those fundamental laws of healing can be applied to ourselves and our society. We can feel the full vital life force within us and become fully alive because we have ignited healing power within us and between us.

The good news is that the healing path is easy and accessible to all of us. Although there are diverse languages and practices of healing in every culture, healing itself requires no specific religious belief. The path of healing doesn't even require another person—remember, nobody else can heal you; they can only help to jump-start your own healing process.

The best way we can foster healing for others is to ensure that we are also making ourselves whole. I wish for you a full realization of your healing potential. Sending you much love, now and always.

ACKNOWLEDGMENTS

I share deep gratitude first to my husband and soulmate, Vikas Srivastava. This book could not have been written without your unwavering support. Even when it has made things hard for you, you have always been there for me. Thank you for all that you do to support me, the family, and the world. I look forward to returning the favor as you write your first book!

Thank you also to my children, Suhani and Akaash, who inspire me daily, keep me honest, and remind me to live life with joy. Being your Mom is definitely the best thing I have ever done and will ever do with my life. I love you more than the universe and will always be here to support you, no matter what.

Thank you to my father, who has been encouraging me to write this book for nearly 20 years! Thank you for believing in me, and thank you and Mom for your unwavering love and support.

Thank you to my second set of parents, Meera and Shabd Srivastava. Not only have you raised an incredible son, you have welcomed me into your family as a third daughter and continue to be an example of love, light, and grace.

Thank you to my brothers in healing, Richard Hammerschlag and David Muehsam, who set upon the Consciousness and Healing Initiative (CHI) journey with me and who continue to offer wholehearted support of our mission—including reading and commenting on parts of this book. Thank you also to Meredith Sprengel, who tirelessly and cheerfully supports our work at CHI.

Thank you to Rachel Lehmann-Haupt—you have been the perfect editor for this book! I'm so glad this project opened your eyes and heart to the power of the biofield.

Thank you to Sounds True and especially Tami Simon—your encouragement is what led me to write this book. Thank you for seeing the value in the biofield.

Lastly, thank you to all my past and present advisors and the ancestors and spirits who continue to guide me. You are the light that illuminates my path, and I am blessed to be a faithful student of your wisdom.

NOTES

Following are the peer-reviewed scientific papers referenced in each chapter.

Introduction

1. Institute for Health Metrics and Evaluation (IHME), *Findings from the Global Burden of Disease Study 2017* (Seattle, WA: IHME, 2018).
2. National Alliance on Mental Illness (NAMI), *Mental Health by the Numbers* (Arlington, VA: NAMI, 2020), nami.org/mhstats.
3. Centers for Disease Control (CDC), *Health and Economic Costs of Chronic Disease* (Atlanta, GA: CDC, 2020), cdc.gov/chronicdisease/about/costs/index.htm.
4. World Health Organization (WHO), *Mental Health Included in the UN Sustainable Development Goals* (Geneva: WHO, 2020), who.int/mental_health /SDGs/en/.

Chapter 1: The Biofield

1 World Health Organization (WHO), *Integrated Chronic Disease Prevention and Control* (Geneva: WHO, 2020), who.int/chp/about/integrated_cd/en/.
2. B. Wang, R. Li, Z. Lu, and Y. Huang, "Does Comorbidity Increase the Risk of Patients with Covid-19: Evidence from Meta-Analysis," *Aging* 12, no. 7 (2020): 6049–6057, doi: 10.18632/aging.103000.
3. R. D. Knaggs and C. Stannard, "Opioid Prescribing: Balancing Overconsumption and Undersupply," *British Journal of Pain* 11, no. 1 (2017): 5, doi: 10.1177/2049463716684055.
4. Society of Actuaries, "Economic Impact of Non-Medical Opioid Use in the United States" (October 2019), soa.org/globalassets/assets/files/resources/research -report/2019/econ-impact-non-medical-opioid-use.pdf.
5. S. Berterame, J. Erthal, J. Thomas, et al., "Use of and Barriers to Access to Opioid Analgesics: A Worldwide, Regional, and National Study," *Lancet* 387, no. 10028 (2016): 1644–1656, doi: 10.1016/S0140-6736(16)00161-6.
6. Drug Policy Alliance, *Drug Overdose* (2020), drugpolicy.org/issues/drug-overdose.
7. "Global, Regional, and National Incidence, Prevalence, and Years Lived with Disability for 354 Diseases and Injuries for 195 Countries and Territories, 1990–2017: A Systematic Analysis for the Global Burden of Disease Study 2017," *Lancet* (2020), thelancet.com/journals/lancet/article/PIIS0140-6736(18)32279-7/fulltext.
8. E. T. Withington, "The History of Medicine," *BMJ* 2 (1912): 659, doi: 10.1136 /bmj.2.2698.659.

9. H. J. Flint, K. P. Scott, P. Louis, and S. H. Duncan, "The Role of the Gut Microbiota in Nutrition and Health," *Nature Reviews Gastroenterology and Hepatology* 9, no. 10 (2012): 577–589, doi: 10.1038/nrgastro.2012.156.

10. "Neuroimmune Communication," *Nature Neuroscience* 20, no. 2 (2017), doi: 10.1038/nn.4496.

11. G. Filipp and A. Szentivanyi, "Anaphylaxis and Nervous System: Part I," *Acta Medica Hungarica* (1952): 2.

12. George F. Soloman, "The Development and History of Psychoneuroimmunology," in *The Link Between Religion and Health: Psychoneuroimmunology and the Faith Factor*, ed. Harold G. Koenig and H. J. Cohen (Oxford, UK: Oxford University Press, 2001).

13. H. Besedovsky, E. Sorkin, D. Felix, et al., "Hypothalamic Changes During the Immune Response," *European Journal of Immunology* (1977), doi: 10.1002/eji.1830070516.

14. R. Ader and N. Cohen, "Behaviorally Conditioned Immunosuppression," *Psychosomatic Medicine* (1975), doi: 10.1097/00006842-197507000-00007.

15. C. B. Pert, M. R. Ruff, R. J. Weber, et al., "Neuropeptides and Their Receptors: A Psychosomatic Network," *Journal of Immunology* (1950).

16. R. Ader, "Historical Perspectives on Psychoneuroimmunology," in *Psychoneuroimmunology, Stress, and Infection*, ed. H. Friedman, T. W. Klein, and A. L. Friedman (Boca Raton, FL: CRC Press, 1995), 1–24.

17. R. Zhu, Z. Sun, C. Li, et al., "Electrical Stimulation Affects Neural Stem Cell Fate and Function in Vitro," *Experimental Neurology* (2019), doi: 10.1016/j.expneurol.2019.112963.

18. M. Newton, K. Peng, and E. Sonera, "Electromechanical Properties of Bone," *International Journal of Engineering Science* (2013).

19. G. Chevalier, S. T. Sinatra, J. L. Oschman, et al., "Earthing: Health Implications of Reconnecting the Human Body to the Earth's Surface Electrons," *Journal of Environmental and Public Health*, doi: 10.1155/2012/291541.

20. C. X. Wang, I. A. Hilburn, D. A. Wu, et al., "Transduction of the Geomagnetic Field as Evidenced from Alpha-Band Activity in the Human Brain," *eNeuro* (2019), doi: 10.1523/ENEURO.0483-18.2019.

21. A. Alabdulgader, R. McCraty, M. Atkinson, et al., "Long-Term Study of Heart Rate Variability Responses to Changes in the Solar and Geomagnetic Environment," *Scientific Reports* (2018), doi: 10.1038/s41598-018-20932-x; J. M. Caswell, M. Singh, and M. A. Persinger, "Simulated Sudden Increase in Geomagnetic Activity and Its Effect on Heart Rate Variability: Experimental Verification of Correlation Studies," *Life Sciences in Space Research* (2016), doi: 10.1016/j.lssr.2016.08.001.

22. M. Levin, "Molecular Bioelectricity: How Endogenous Voltage Potentials Control Cell Behavior and Instruct Pattern Regulation in Vivo," *Molecular Biology of the Cell* 25, no. 24 (2014): 3835–3850, doi: 10.1091/mbc.E13-12-0708.

23. M. Levin, "Reprogramming Cells and Tissue Patterning via Bioelectrical Pathways: Molecular Mechanisms and Biomedical Opportunities," *Wiley Interdisciplinary Reviews: Systems Biology and Medicine* 5, no. 6 (2013): 657–676, doi: 10.1002/wsbm.1236.

24. N. Lipsman, Y. Meng, A. J. Bethune, et al., "Blood-Brain Barrier Opening in Alzheimer's Disease Using MR-Guided Focused Ultrasound," *Nature Communications* 9, no. 1 (2018): 1–8, doi: 10.1038/s41467-018-04529-6; D. Muehsam, G. Chevalier, T. Barsotti, et al., "An Overview of Biofield Devices," *Global Advances in Health and Medicine* 4, Suppl. (2015): 42–51, doi: 10.7453/gahmj.2015.022.suppl.

Chapter 2: The Search Begins

1. J. D. Long, *Jainism: An Introduction* (New York: Macmillan, 2009).

Chapter 3: Consciousness

1. J. Daubenmier, D. Chopra, S. Jain, et al., "Indo-Tibetan Philosophical and Medical Systems: Perspectives on the Biofield," *Global Advances in Health and Medicine* (2015), doi: 10.7453/gahmj.2015.026.suppl.

2. E. Laszlo, J. Houston, and L. Dossey, *What Is Consciousness? Three Sages Look Behind the Veil* (New York: SelectBooks, 2016).

3. C. G. Jung, *The Archetypes and the Collective Unconscious*, trans. R. F. C. Hull (Princeton, NJ: Princeton University Press, 1959).

4. P. Livingston, "Experience and Structure: Philosophical History and the Problem of Consciousness," *Journal of Consciousness Studies* (2002).

5. D. J. Chalmers, "Facing Up to the Problem of Consciousness: The Character of Consciousness," *Journal of Consciousness Studies* 2, no. 3 (1995): 200–219, doi: 10.1093/acprof.

6. P. Churchland, *Touching a Nerve: Our Brains, Our Selves* (New York: Norton, 2013).

7. D. J. Chalmers, *The Character of Consciousness* (Oxford, UK: Oxford University Press, 2010).

8. S. Brier, "How Peircean Semiotic Philosophy Connects Western Science with Eastern Emptiness Ontology," *Progress in Biophysics and Molecular Biology* (2017), doi: 10.1016/j.pbiomolbio.2017.08.011.

9. J. Shear, "Eastern Methods for Investigating Mind and Consciousness," in *The Blackwell Companion to Consciousness* (London: Blackwell, 2007), doi: 10.1002/9780470751466.ch55.

10. C. S. Peirce, *Collected Papers of C. S. Peirce, 1931–1958* (Cambridge, MA: Harvard University Press, 1960).

11. Daubenmier, Chopra, Jain, et al., "Indo-Tibetan Philosophical and Medical Systems"; W. M. Indich, *Consciousness in Advaita Vedanta* (Delhi: Motilal Banarsidass, 1995); R. E. Hume, *The Thirteen Principal Upanishads: Translated from the Sanskrit with an Outline of the Philosophy of the Upanishads and an Annotated Bibliography*, trans. H. Milford (Oxford, UK: Oxford University Press, 1921).

12. H. Wahbeh, A. Sagher, W. Back, et al., "A Systematic Review of Transcendent States Across Meditation and Contemplative Traditions," *Explore* (2017), doi: 10.1016 /j.explore.2017.07.007.

13. P. Yogananda, *Autobiography of a Yogi* (New York: Philosophical Library, 1946).

14. E. F. Bryant, *The Yoga Sutras of Patanjali: A New Edition, Translation, and Commentary* (New York: North Point Press, 2015); S. Krishnananda, *The Mandukya Upanishad: An Exposition* (Rishikesh, India: Divine Life Society, 1997); G. Samuel and J. Johnston, eds., *Religion and the Subtle Body in Asia and the West: Between Mind and Body* (London: Routledge, 2013).

Chapter 4: Subtle Bodies and the "Stain of Vitalism"

1. B. Rubik, "The Biofield Hypothesis: Its Biophysical Basis and Role in Medicine," *Journal of Alternative and Complementary Medicine* (2003), doi: 10.1089/10755530260511711.

2. A. C. Logan and E. M. Selhub, "*Vis Medicatrix naturae*: Does Nature 'Minister to the Mind'?" *BioPsychoSocial Medicine* 6, no. 1 (2012): 11, doi: 10.1186/1751 -0759-6-11.

3. D. Frawley, *Inner Tantric Yoga: Working with the Universal Shakti—Secrets of Mantras, Deities, and Meditation* (Detroit: Lotus, 2009).

4. M. Prasad, ed., *The Taittiriya Upanishad: With the Original Text in Sanskrit and Roman Transliteration* (Columbia, MO: South Asia Books, 1994).

5. S. Krishnananda, *The Mandukya Upanishad: An Exposition* (Rishikesh, India: Divine Life Society, 1997).

6. P. Prajnanananda, *Jnana Sankalini Tantra* (Delhi: Motilal Banarsidass, 2010); S. N. Saraswati, *Prana, Pranayama, Prana Vidya* (Munger, India: Yoga Publications Trust, 1994).

7. T. Umasvati, *That Which Is: Tattvartha Sutra* (Fremont, CA: Jain, 2002); B. Gerke, "On the 'Subtle Body' and 'Circulation' in Tibetan Medicine," in *Religion and the Subtle Body in Asia and the West*, ed. G. Samuel and J. Johnston (London: Routledge, 2013), 97–113; G. Samuel and J. Johnston, eds., *Religion and the Subtle Body in Asia and the West: Between Mind and Body* (London: Routledge, 2013); S. S. Saraswati and N. Nikolić, *Kundalini Tantra* (Munger, India: Bihar School of Yoga, 1984).

8. J. Daubenmier, D. Chopra, S. Jain, et al., "Indo-Tibetan Philosophical and Medical Systems: Perspectives on the Biofield," *Global Advances in Health and Medicine* (2015), doi: 10.7453/gahmj.2015.026.suppl.

9. N. L. Kachhara, "Philosophy of Mind: A Jain Perspective," *US-China Education Review* (2011).

10. Krishnananda, *Mandukya Upanishad*; R. E. Hume, *The Thirteen Principal Upanishads: Translated from the Sanskrit with an Outline of the Philosophy of the Upanishads and an Annotated Bibliography,* trans. H. Milford (Oxford, UK: Oxford University Press, 1921).

11. R. Svoboda and A. Lade, *Tao and Dharma: Chinese Medicine and Ayurveda* (Detroit: Lotus, 1995); M. Greenwood, "Acupuncture and the Chakras," *Medical Acupuncture* 17, no. 3 (2006): 27–32.

12. A. A. Bailey, *The Seventh Ray: Revealer of the New Age* (New York: Lucis, 1995); S. S. Goswami, *Layayoga: The Definitive Guide to the Chakras and Kundalini* (Rochester, VT: Inner Traditions, 1999).

13. V. Ogay, K. H. Bae, K. W. Kim, et al., "Comparison of the Characteristic Features of Bonghan Ducts, Blood, and Lymphatic Capillaries," *Journal of Acupuncture and Meridian Studies* 2, no. 2 (2009): 107–117, doi: 10.1016/S2005-2901(09)60042-X; K.-S. Soh, "Bonghan Circulatory System as an Extension of Acupuncture Meridians," *Journal of Acupuncture and Meridian Studies* 2, no. 2 (2009): 93–106, doi: 10.1016/S2005-2901(09)60041-8.

14. R. Bhargava, M. G. Gogate, and J. F. Mascarenhas, "Autonomic Responses to Breath Holding and Its Variations Following Pranayama," *Indian Journal of Physiology and Pharmacology* 32, no. 4 (1988): 257–264; T. Pramanik, H. O. Sharma, S. Mishra, et al., "Immediate Effect of Slow Pace Bhastrika Pranayama on Blood Pressure and Heart Rate," *Journal of Alternative and Complementary Medicine* 15, no. 3 (2009): 293–295, doi: 10.1089/acm.2008.0440.

15. Daubenmier, Chopra, Jain, et al., "Indo-Tibetan Philosophical and Medical Systems"; S. Deane, "Lung, Mind, and Mental Health: The Notion of 'Wind' in Tibetan Conceptions of Mind and Mental Illness," *Journal of Religion and Health* (2019), doi: 10.1007/s10943-019-00775-0; M. Epstein and L. Rapgay, "Mind, Disease, and Health in Tibetan Medicine," in *Healing East and West: Ancient Wisdom and Modern Psychology*, ed. A. A. Sheikh and K. S. Sheikh (London: Wiley, 1989), doi: 10.1163/1568538054253375; R. Yoeli-Tlalim, "Tibetan 'Wind' and 'Wind' Illnesses: Towards a Multicultural Approach to Health and Illness," *Studies in History and Philosophy of Science, Part C: Studies in History and Philosophy of Biological and Biomedical Sciences* 41, no. 4 (2010), doi: 10.1016/j.shpsc.2010.10.005.

16. G. F. Solomon and R. H. Moos, "Emotions, Immunity, and Disease: A Speculative Theoretical Integration," *Archives of General Psychiatry* 11, no. 6 (1964): 657–674, doi: 10.1001/archpsyc.1964.01720300087011.

17. D. F. Strauss, "Hylozoism and Hylomorphism: A Lasting Legacy of Greek Philosophy," *Phronimon* (2019), doi: 10.25159/2413-3086/2211.

18. G. Federspil and N. Sicolo, "The Nature of Life in the History of Medical and Philosophic Thinking," *American Journal of Nephrology* (1994), doi: 10.1159/000168745.

19. R. P. Aulie, "Caspar Friedrich Wolff and His 'Theoria Generationis,' 1759," *Journal of the History of Medicine and Allied Sciences* (1961), doi: 10.1093/jhmas/XVI.2.124.

20. E. Kinne-Saffran and R. K. Kinne, "Vitalism and Synthesis of Urea: From Friedrich Wöhler to Hans A. Krebs," *American Journal of Nephrology* (1999): 13463.

21. J. H. Brooke, "Wöhler's Urea and Its Vital Force? A Verdict from the Chemists," *Ambix* 15, no. 2 (1968): 84–114, doi: 10.1179/amb.1968.15.2.84; R. L. Numbers and K. Kampourakis, *Newton's Apple and Other Myths about Science* (Cambridge, MA: Harvard University Press, 2015).

22. F. Crick, *Of Molecules and Men* (London: Prometheus, 2004).

23. S. Oyama, "Biologists Behaving Badly: Vitalism and the Language of Language," *History and Philosophy of the Life Sciences* 32, nos. 2–3 (2010): 401–423.

24. L. Hilton, S. Hempel, B. A. Ewing, et al., "Mindfulness Meditation for Chronic Pain: Systematic Review and Meta-Analysis," *Annals of Behavioral Medicine* 51, no. 2 (2017): 199–213, doi: 10.1007/s12160-016-9844-2; M. C. Pascoe, D. R. Thompson, and C. F. Ski, "Yoga, Mindfulness-Based Stress Reduction, and Stress-Related Physiological Measures: A Meta-Analysis," *Psychoneuroendocrinology* 86 (2017): 152–168, doi: 10.1016/j.psyneuen.2017.08.008; H. Cramer, R. Lauche, P. Klose, et al., "Yoga for Improving Health-Related Quality of Life, Mental Health, and Cancer-Related Symptoms in Women Diagnosed with Breast Cancer," *Cochrane Database of Systematic Reviews* 1, no. CD010802 (2017), doi: 10.1002/14651858.CD010802.pub2; S. Jain and P. J. Mills, "Biofield Therapies: Helpful or Full of Hype? A Best Evidence Synthesis," *International Journal of Behavioral Medicine* 17 (2010), doi: 10.1007/s12529-009-9062-4.

25. C. Vieten, H. Wahbeh, B. R. Cahn, et al., "Future Directions in Meditation Research: Recommendations for Expanding the Field of Contemplative Science," *PLoS One* 13, no. 11 (2018), doi: 10.1371/journal.pone.0205740.

26. "Energy Healing Sparks Debate," *Chicago Tribune,* December 11, 2011, chicagotribune.com/lifestyles/ct-xpm-2011-12-11-ct-met-nccam-energy-healing-20111211-story.html.

Chapter 5: Can We Heal Ourselves? The Truth about Placebos

1. A. J. M. De Craen, T. J. Kaptchuk, J. G. P. Tijssen, et al., "Placebos and Placebo Effects in Medicine: Historical Overview," *Journal of the Royal Society of Medicine* 92, no. 10 (1999): 511–515, doi: 10.1177/014107689909201005.

2. D. Forrest, "Mesmer," *International Journal of Clinical and Experimental Hypnosis* 50, no. 4 (2002): 295–308.

3. B. Franklin, L. Majault, J.-S. B. Sallin, et al., "Report of the Commissioners Charged by the King with the Examination of Animal Magnetism," *International Journal of Clinical and Experimental Hypnosis* 50, no. 4 (2002): 332–363, doi: 10.1080/00207140208410109.

4. I. Kirsch and G. Sapirstein, "Listening to Prozac but Hearing Placebo: A Meta-Analysis of Antidepressant Medication," *Prevention and Treatment* 1, no. 2 (1998), doi: 10.1037/1522-3736.1.1.12a.

5. I. Kirsch, T. J. Moore, A. Scoboria, et al., "The Emperor's New Drugs: An Analysis of Antidepressant Medication Data Submitted to the U.S. Food and Drug

Administration," *Prevention and Treatment* 5, no. 1 (2002), doi: 10.1037/1522-3736.5.1.523a.

6. I. Kirsch, "Antidepressants and the Placebo Effect," *Journal of Psychology* 222, no. 3 (2014): 128–134, doi: 10.1027/2151-2604/a000176.

7. L. Colloca and F. Benedetti, "Science and Society: Placebos and Painkillers—Is Mind as Real as Matter?" *Nature Reviews Neuroscience* 6, no. 7 (2005): 545–552, doi: 10.1038/nrn1705.

8. J. J. Cragg, F. M. Warner, N. B. Finnerup, et al., "Meta-Analysis of Placebo Responses in Central Neuropathic Pain: Impact of Subject, Study, and Pain Characteristics," *Pain* 157, no. 3 (2016): 530–540, doi: 10.1097/j.pain.0000000000000431.

9. L. Vase, J. L. Riley, and D. D. Price, "A Comparison of Placebo Effects in Clinical Analgesic Trials Versus Studies of Placebo Analgesia," *Pain* 99, no. 3 (2002): 443–452, doi: 10.1016/S0304-3959(02)00205-1.

10. K. Wartolowska, A. Judge, S. Hopewell, et al., "Use of Placebo Controls in the Evaluation of Surgery: Systematic Review," *BMJ* 348 (2014), doi: 10.1136/bmj.g3253.

11. W. B. Jonas, C. Crawford, L. Colloca, et al., "To What Extent Are Surgery and Invasive Procedures Effective Beyond a Placebo Response? A Systematic Review with Meta-Analysis of Randomised, Sham Controlled Trials," *BMJ Open* 5, no. 12 (2015), doi: 10.1136/bmjopen-2015-009655.

12. T. J. Kaptchuk, E. Friedlander, J. M. Kelley, et al., "Placebos Without Deception: A Randomized Controlled Trial in Irritable Bowel Syndrome," *PLoS One* 5, no. 12 (2010), doi: 10.1371/journal.pone.0015591.

13. C. Carvalho, J. M. Caetano, L. Cunha, et al., "Open-Label Placebo Treatment in Chronic Low Back Pain," *Pain* 157, no. 12 (2016): 2766–2772, doi: 10.1097/j.pain.0000000000000700; S. Ballou, T. J. Kaptchuk, W. Hirsch, et al., "Open-Label Versus Double-Blind Placebo Treatment in Irritable Bowel Syndrome: Study Protocol for a Randomized Controlled Trial," *Trials* 18, no. 1 (2017), doi: 10.1186/s13063-017-1964-x.

14. T. W. Hoenemeyer, T. J. Kaptchuk, T. S. Mehta, et al., "Open-Label Placebo Treatment for Cancer-Related Fatigue: A Randomized-Controlled Clinical Trial," *Scientific Reports* 8, no. 1 (2018): 2784, doi: 10.1038/s41598-018-20993-y.

15. T. D. Wager, "Placebo-Induced Changes in fMRI in the Anticipation and Experience of Pain," *Science* 303, no. 5661 (2004): 1162–1167, doi: 10.1126/science.1093065.

16. D. D. Price, D. G. Finniss, and F. Benedetti, "A Comprehensive Review of the Placebo Effect: Recent Advances and Current Thought," *Annual Review of Psychology* (2008), doi: 10.1146/annurev.psych.59.113006.095941.

17. F. Benedetti, L. Colloca, E. Torre, et al., "Placebo-Responsive Parkinson Patients Show Decreased Activity in Single Neurons of Subthalamic Nucleus," *Nature Neuroscience* 7, no. 6 (2004): 587–588, doi: 10.1038/nn1250.

18. N. Shetty, J. H. Friedman, K. Kieburtz, et al., "The Placebo Response in Parkinson's Disease: Parkinson Study Group," *Clinical Neuropharmacology* 22, no. 4 (1999): 207–212.

19. R. de la Fuente-Fernández, A. G. Phillips, M. Zamburlini, et al., "Dopamine Release in Human Ventral Striatum and Expectation of Reward," *Behavioural Brain Research* (2002), doi: 10.1016/S0166-4328(02)00130-4.

20. A. Keitel, S. Ferrea, M. Südmeyer, et al., "Expectation Modulates the Effect of Deep Brain Stimulation on Motor and Cognitive Function in Tremor-Dominant Parkinson's Disease," *PLoS One* 8, no. 12 (2013), e81878, doi: 10.1371/journal .pone.0081878; A. Pollo, E. Torre, L. Lopiano, et al., "Expectation Modulates the Response to Subthalamic Nucleus Stimulation in Parkinsonian Patients," *NeuroReport* (2002), doi: 10.1097/00001756-200208070-00006; R. de la Fuente-Fernández, "Uncovering the Hidden Placebo Effect in Deep-Brain Stimulation for Parkinson's Disease," *Parkinsonism and Related Disorders* 10, no. 3 (2004): 125–127, doi: 10.1016/j.parkreldis.2003.10.003.

21. E. Frisaldi, E. Carlino, M. Lanotte, et al., "Characterization of the Thalamic-Subthalamic Circuit Involved in the Placebo Response Through Single-Neuron Recording in Parkinson Patients," *Cortex* 60 (2014): 3–9.

22. M. Amanzio and F. Benedetti, "Neuropharmacological Dissection of Placebo Analgesia: Expectation-Activated Opioid Systems Versus Conditioning-Activated Specific Subsystems," *Journal of Neuroscience* 19, no. 1 (1999): 484–494, doi: 10.1038/nrn3465.

23. L. Colloca, "The Placebo Effect in Pain Therapies," *Annual Review of Pharmacology and Toxicology* 59 (2019): 191–211, doi: 10.1146/annurev-pharmtox-010818-021542.

24. K. Meissner and K. Linde, "Are Blue Pills Better Than Green? How Treatment Features Modulate Placebo Effects," in *International Review of Neurobiology, vol. 139: Neurobiology of the Placebo Effect*, Part 2, ed. L. Colloca (San Diego: Academic Press, 2018), 357–378, doi: 10.1016/bs.irn.2018.07.014.

25. E. R. C. M. Huisman, E. Morales, J. van Hoof, et al., "Healing Environment: A Review of the Impact of Physical Environmental Factors on Users," *Building and Environment* 58 (2012): 70–80, doi: 10.1016/j.buildenv.2012.06.016; E. M. Sternberg, *Healing Spaces* (Cambridge, MA: Harvard University Press, 2009).

26. B. D. Darnall and L. Colloca, "Optimizing Placebo and Minimizing Nocebo to Reduce Pain, Catastrophizing, and Opioid Use: A Review of the Science and an Evidence-Informed Clinical Toolkit," *International Review of Neurobiology* 139 (2018): 129–157, doi: 10.1016/bs.irn.2018.07.022.

27. A.-K. Bräscher, M. Witthöft, and S. Becker, "The Underestimated Significance of Conditioning in Placebo Hypoalgesia and Nocebo Hyperalgesia," *Pain Research and Management* 2018 (2018): 6841985, doi: 10.1155/2018/6841985.

28. M. Blasini, N. Peiris, T. Wright, et al., "The Role of Patient-Practitioner Relationships in Placebo and Nocebo Phenomena," *International Review of Neurobiology* 139 (2018): 211–231, doi: 10.1016/bs.irn.2018.07.033.

29. D. Rakel, B. Barrett, Z. Zhang, et al., "Perception of Empathy in the Therapeutic Encounter: Effects on the Common Cold," *Patient Education and Counseling* 85, no. 3 (2011): 390–397.

30. S. A. Green, "Surgeons and Shamans: The Placebo Value of Ritual," *Clinical Orthopaedics and Related Research* 450 (2006): 249–254, doi: 10.1097/01.blo .0000224044.69592.65; J. S. Welch, "Ritual in Western Medicine and Its Role in Placebo Healing," *Journal of Religion and Health* 42, no. 1 (2003): 21–33, doi: 10.1023/A:1022260610761.

31. D. G. Finniss, T. J. Kaptchuk, F. Miller, et al., "Placebo Effects: Biological, Clinical, and Ethical Advances," *Lancet* 375, no. 9715 (2018): 686–695, doi: 10.1016 /S0140-6736(09)61706-2.

32. Jonas, Crawford, Colloca, et al., "To What Extent Are Surgery and Invasive Procedures Effective Beyond a Placebo Response?"

Chapter 6: Can We Heal Ourselves? Mind-Body Therapies

1. E. F. Bryant, *The Yoga Sutras of Patanjali: A New Edition, Translation, and Commentary* (New York: North Point Press, 2015).

2. G. Jha et al., *The Yoga-Darśana: The Sutras of Patañjali with the Bhāsya of Vyasa* (Rajaram Tukaram Tatya, 1907); G. Feuerstein, *The Yoga Tradition: Its History, Literature, Philosophy, and Practice* (Los Angeles: SCB Distributors, 2012).

3. P. Yogananda, *The Yoga of Jesus* (Los Angeles: Self-Realization Fellowship, 2009); J. A. O'Brien, *Meeting of Mystic Paths: Christianity and Yoga* (Saint Paul, MN: Yes International, 1996).

4. A. Bussing, T. Ostermann, R. Ludtke, et al., *Effects of Yoga Interventions on Pain and Pain-Associated Disability: A Meta-Analysis* (York, UK: Centre for Reviews and Dissemination, 2012).

5. A. C. Skelly, R. Chou, J. R. Dettori, et al., *Noninvasive Nonpharmacological Treatment for Chronic Pain: A Systematic Review Update* (Rockville, MD: Agency for Healthcare Research and Quality, 2020).

6. J. S. Armer and S. K. Lutgendorf, "The Impact of Yoga on Fatigue in Cancer Survivorship: A Meta-Analysis," *JNCI Cancer Spectrum* 4, no. 2 (2020): pkz098, doi: 10.1093/jncics/pkz098.

7. M. Shohani, F. Kazemi, S. Rahmati, et al., "The Effect of Yoga on the Quality of Life and Fatigue in Patients with Multiple Sclerosis: A Systematic Review and Meta-Analysis of Randomized Clinical Trials," *Complementary Therapies in Clinical Practice* 39 (2020): 101087, doi: 10.1016/j.ctcp.2020.101087.

8. D. Anheyer, P. Klose, R. Lauche, et al., "Yoga for Treating Headaches: A Systematic Review and Meta-Analysis," *Journal of General Internal Medicine* 35, no. 3 (2020): 846–854, doi: 10.1007/s11606-019-05413-9.

9. H. Cramer, W. Peng, and R. Lauche, "Yoga for Menopausal Symptoms: A Systematic Review and Meta-Analysis," *Maturitas* 109 (2018): 13–25, doi: 10.1016/j.maturitas.2017.12.005.

10. H. Cramer, D. Anheyer, R. Lauche, et al., "A Systematic Review of Yoga for Major Depressive Disorder," *Journal of Affective Disorders* 213 (2017): 70–77; M. Balasubramaniam, S. Telles, and P. M. Doraiswamy, "Yoga on Our Minds: A Systematic Review of Yoga for Neuropsychiatric Disorders," *Frontiers in Psychiatry* 3 (2013): 117.

11. G. Kirkwood, H. Rampes, V. Tuffrey, et al., "Yoga for Anxiety: A Systematic Review of the Research Evidence," *British Journal of Sports Medicine* 39, no. 12 (2005): 884–891, doi: 10.1136/bjsm.2005.018069.

12. M. Kuppusamy, D. Kamaldeen, R. Pitani, et al., "Effects of Bhramari Pranayama on Health: A Systematic Review," *Journal of Traditional Complementary Medicine* 8, no. 1 (2017): 11–16, doi: 10.1016/j.jtcme.2017.02.003; T. Pramanik, H. O. Sharma, S. Mishra, et al., "Immediate Effect of Slow Pace Bhastrika Pranayama on Blood Pressure and Heart Rate," *Journal of Alternative and Complementary Medicine* 15, no. 3 (2009): 293–295; R. Bhargava, M. G. Gogate, and J. F. Mascarenhas, "Autonomic Responses to Breath Holding and Its Variations Following Pranayama," *Indian Journal of Physiology and Pharmacology* 32, no. 4 (1988): 8.

13. A. E. Holland, C. J. Hill, A. Y. Jones, et al., "Breathing Exercises for Chronic Obstructive Pulmonary Disease," *Cochrane Database of Systematic Reviews,* doi: 10.1002/14651858.CD008250.pub2.

14. J. J. Allen, "Characteristics of Users and Reported Effects of the Wim Hof Method: A Mixed-Methods Study" (2018), purl.utwente.nl/essays/76839; O. Muzik, K. T. Reilly, and V. A. Diwadkar, "Brain over Body: A Study on the Willful Regulation of Autonomic Function during Cold Exposure," *NeuroImage* 172 (2018): 632–641.

15. T. Chetwynd, *Zen and the Kingdom of Heaven: Reflections on the Tradition of Meditation in Christianity and Zen Buddhism* (New York: Simon and Schuster, 2001); H. Eifring, *Meditation in Judaism, Christianity, and Islam: Cultural Histories* (London: A & C Black, 2013); T. Frederick and K. M. White, "Mindfulness, Christian Devotion Meditation, Surrender, and Worry," *Mental Health, Religion, and Culture* 18, no. 10 (2015): 850–858, doi: 10.1080/13674676.2015.1107892.

16. A. Burke, C. N. Lam, B. Stussman, et al., "Prevalence and Patterns of Use of Mantra, Mindfulness, and Spiritual Meditation among Adults in the United States," *BMC Complementary and Alternative Medicine* 17, no. 1 (2017): 316, doi: 10.1186 /s12906-017-1827-8.

17. L. Larkey, R. Jahnke, J. Etnier, et al., "Meditative Movement as a Category of Exercise: Implications for Research," *Journal of Physical Activity and Health* 6, no. 2 (2009): 230–238; P. Posadzki and S. Jacques, "Tai Chi and Meditation: A Conceptual (Re)Synthesis?" *Journal of Holistic Nursing* 27, no. 2 (2009): 103–114, doi: 10.1177/0898010108330807; R. Lauche, P. M. Wayne, G. Dobos, et al., "Prevalence, Patterns, and Predictors of T'ai Chi and Qigong Use in the United States: Results of a Nationally Representative Survey," *Journal of Alternative and Complementary Medicine* 22, no. 4 (2016): 336–342, doi: 10.1089/acm.2015.0356.

18. C. Titmuss, "Is There a Corporate Takeover of the Mindfulness Industry? An Exploration of Western Mindfulness in the Public and Private Sector," in *Handbook of Mindfulness: Culture, Context, and Social Engagement*, ed. R. E. Purser, D. Forbes, and A. Burke (New York: Springer, 2016), 181–194, doi: 10.1007/978-3 -319-44019-4_13; P. Moloney, "Mindfulness: The Bottled Water of the Therapy Industry," in *Handbook of Mindfulness: Culture, Context, and Social Engagement*, ed. R. E. Purser, D. Forbes, and A. Burke (New York: Springer, 2016), 269–292, doi: 10.1007/978-3-319-44019-4_18.

19. S. Jain, S. L. Shapiro, S. Swanick, et al., "A Randomized Controlled Trial of Mindfulness Meditation Versus Relaxation Training: Effects on Distress, Positive States of Mind, Rumination, and Distraction," *Annals of Behavioral Medicine* (2007), doi: 10.1207/s15324796abm3301_2; J. L. Kristeller, "Mindfulness Meditation," in *Principles and Practice of Stress Management*, 3rd ed., ed. P. M. Lehrer, R. L. Woolfolk, and W. E. Sime (New York: Guilford, 2007), 393–427.

20. J. Daubenmier, D. Chopra, S. Jain, et al., "Indo-Tibetan Philosophical and Medical Systems: Perspectives on the Biofield," *Global Advances in Health and Medicine* (2015), doi: 10.7453/gahmj.2015.026.suppl.

21. L. Hilton, S. Hempel, B. A. Ewing, et al., "Mindfulness Meditation for Chronic Pain: Systematic Review and Meta-Analysis," *Annals of Behavioral Medicine* 51, no. 2 (2017): 199–213, doi: 10.1007/s12160-016-9844-2.

22. M. Goyal, S. Singh, E. M. S. Sibinga, et al., "Meditation Programs for Psychological Stress and Well-Being: A Systematic Review and Meta-Analysis," *JAMA Internal Medicine* (2014), doi: 10.1001/jamainternmed.2013.13018.

23. M. Janssen, Y. Heerkens, W. Kuijer, et al., "Effects of Mindfulness-Based Stress Reduction on Employees' Mental Health: A Systematic Review," *PLoS One* 13, no. 1 (2018): e0191332, doi: 10.1371/journal.pone.0191332.

24. J. Piet, H. Würtzen, and R. Zachariae, "The Effect of Mindfulness-Based Therapy on Symptoms of Anxiety and Depression in Adult Cancer Patients and Survivors: A Systematic Review and Meta-Analysis," *Journal of Consulting and Clinical Psychology* 80, no. 6 (2012): 1007.

25. Y.-Y. Tang, B. K. Hölzel, and M. I. Posner, "The Neuroscience of Mindfulness Meditation," *Nature Reviews Neuroscience* 16, no. 4 (2015): 213–225, doi: 10.1038 /nrn3916.

26. D. S. Black and G. M. Slavich, "Mindfulness Meditation and the Immune System: A Systematic Review of Randomized Controlled Trials," *Annals of the New York Academy of Sciences* 1373, no. 1 (2016): 13–24, doi: 10.1111/nyas.12998.

27. W. Ishak, R. Nikravesh, S. Lederer, et al., "Burnout in Medical Students: A Systematic Review," *Clinical Teacher* 10, no. 4 (2013): 242–245, doi: 10.1111/tct.12014.

28. S. Nolen-Hoeksema, "The Role of Rumination in Depressive Disorders and Mixed Anxiety/Depressive Symptoms," *Journal of Abnormal Psychology* 109, no. 3 (2000): 504.

29. M.-R. Ungunmerr, "To Be Listened to in Her Teaching: Dadirri—Inner Deep Listening and Quiet Still Awareness," *EarthSong Journal: Perspectives in Ecology, Spirituality, and Education* 3, no. 4 (2017): 14; H. Eifring, *Asian Traditions of Meditation* (Honolulu: University of Hawaii Press, 2016); D. P. Broww, "A Model for the Levels of Concentrative Meditation," *International Journal of Clinical and Experimental Hypnosis* 25, no. 4 (1977): 236–273, doi: 10.1080/00207147708415984.

30. T. Keating, *Centering Prayer in Daily Life and Ministry* (New York: Bloomsbury, 1997).

31. V. M. N. Ariyadhamma, "Anapana Sati Meditation on Breathing," in *Bodhi Leaves Publications* (Onalaska, WA: Pariyatti, 1988), 115; W. Shih, "The Technique for Equanimity of Mind Through the Meditation Practice of Anapana Smrti," International Conference on Buddhist Education, Institute for Sino Indian Buddhist Studies (1994), 92; M. T. Treadway and S. W. Lazar, "The Neurobiology of Mindfulness," in *Clinical Handbook of Mindfulness*, ed. F. Didonna (New York: Springer, 2009), 45–57, doi: 10.1007/978-0-387-09593-6_4.

32. A. Lutz, J. D. Dunne, and R. J. Davidson, "Meditation and the Neuroscience of Consciousness," in *The Cambridge Handbook of Consciousness* (Cambridge, UK: Cambridge University Press, 2007), 499–555.

33. R. S. Bucknell, "Reinterpreting the Jhānas," *Journal of the International Association of Buddhist Studies* (1993): 375–409.

34. J. W. Anderson, C. Liu, and R. J. Kryscio, "Blood Pressure Response to Transcendental Meditation: A Meta-Analysis," *American Journal of Hypertension* 21, no. 3 (2008): 310–316, doi: 10.1038/ajh.2007.65; S. L. Ooi, M. Giovino, and S. C. Pak, "Transcendental Meditation for Lowering Blood Pressure: An Overview of Systematic Reviews and Meta-Analyses," *Complementary Therapies in Medicine* 34 (2017): 26–34, doi: 10.1016/j.ctim.2017.07.008.

35. M. B. Ospina, K. Bond, M. Karkhaneh, et al., "Meditation Practices for Health: State of the Research," *Evidence Report/Technology Assessment* 155 (2007): 1–263.

36. L. Bernardi, P. Sleight, G. Bandinelli, et al., "Effect of Rosary Prayer and Yoga Mantras on Autonomic Cardiovascular Rhythms: Comparative Study," *BMJ* 323, no. 7327 (2001): 1446–1449, doi: 10.1136/bmj.323.7327.1446.

37. X. Chen, J. Cui, R. Li, et al., "Dao Yin (a.k.a. Qigong): Origin, Development, Potential Mechanisms, and Clinical Applications," *Evidence-Based Complementary and Alternative Medicine* (October 2019), doi: 10.1155/2019/3705120.

38. R. Walsh, *The World's Great Wisdom: Timeless Teachings from Religions and Philosophies* (Albany: State University of New York Press, 2014).

39. D. Frawley, *Mantra Yoga and the Primal Sound: Secrets of Seed (Bija) Mantras* (Detroit: Lotus, 2010).

40. K. Cohen, *The Way of Qigong: The Art and Science of Chinese Energy Healing* (New York: Ballantine, 1999).

41. Y. Guo, P. Qiu, and T. Liu, "Tai Ji Quan: An Overview of Its History, Health Benefits, and Cultural Value," *Journal of Sport and Health Science* 3, no. 1 (2014): 3–8, doi: 10.1016/j.jshs.2013.10.004.

42. R. Lauche, W. Peng, C. Ferguson, et al., "Efficacy of Tai Chi and Qigong for the Prevention of Stroke and Stroke Risk Factors: A Systematic Review with Meta-Analysis," *Medicine* 96, no. 45 (2017): e8517, doi: 10.1097 /MD.0000000000008517.

43. C. Wang, J. P. Collet, and J. Lau, "The Effect of Tai Chi on Health Outcomes in Patients with Chronic Conditions: A Systematic Review," *Archives of Internal Medicine* 164, no. 5 (2004): 493–501, doi: 10.1001/archinte.164.5.493.

44. R. Song, W. Grabowska, M. Park, et al., "The Impact of Tai Chi and Qigong Mind-Body Exercises on Motor and Non-Motor Function and Quality of Life in Parkinson's Disease: A Systematic Review and Meta-Analysis," *Parkinsonism and Related Disorders* 41 (2017): 3–13, doi: 10.1016/j.parkreldis.2017.05.019.

45. Y. Zeng, X. Xie, and A. S. K. Cheng, "Qigong or Tai Chi in Cancer Care: An Updated Systematic Review and Meta-Analysis," *Current Oncology Reports* 21, no. 6 (2019): 48, doi: 10.1007/s11912-019-0786-2.

46. S. Song, J. Yu, Y. Ruan, et al., "Ameliorative Effects of Tai Chi on Cancer-Related Fatigue: A Meta-Analysis of Randomized Controlled Trials," *Supportive Care in Cancer* 26, no. 7 (2018): 2091–2102, doi: 10.1007/s00520-018-4136-y.

47. X. Ni, R. J. Chan, P. Yates, et al., "The Effects of Tai Chi on Quality of Life of Cancer Survivors: A Systematic Review and Meta-Analysis," *Supportive Care in Cancer* 27, no. 10 (2019): 3701–3716, doi: 10.1007/s00520-019-04911-0; Y. Zeng, T. Luo, H. Xie, et al., "Health Benefits of Qigong or Tai Chi for Cancer Patients: A Systematic Review and Meta-Analysis," *Complementary Therapies in Medicine* 22, no. 1 (2014): 173–186, doi: 10.1016/j.ctim.2013.11.010.

48. R. T. H. Ho, C.-W. Wang, S.-M. Ng, et al., "The Effect of T'ai Chi Exercise on Immunity and Infections: A Systematic Review of Controlled Trials," *Journal of Alternative and Complementary Medicine* 19, no. 5 (2013): 389–396, doi: 10.1089 /acm.2011.0593.

49. A. M. Alenazi, M. M. Alshehri, J. C. Hoover, et al., "The Effect of T'ai Chi Exercise on Lipid Profiles: A Systematic Review and Meta-Analysis of Randomized Clinical Trials," *Journal of Alternative and Complementary Medicine* 24, no. 3 (2018): 220–230, doi: 10.1089/acm.2017.0104.

50. N. Morgan, M. R. Irwin, M. Chung, et al., "The Effects of Mind-Body Therapies on the Immune System: Meta-Analysis," *PLoS One* 9, no. 7 (2014): e100903, doi: 10.1371/journal.pone.0100903.

51. S. Jain, J. Bower, and M. R. Irwin, "Psychoneuroimmunology of Fatigue and Sleep Disturbance: The Role of Pro-Inflammatory Cytokines," in *The Oxford Handbook of Psychoneuroimmunology*, ed. S. C. Segerstrom (Oxford, UK: Oxford University Press, 2012); E. N. Benveniste, "Inflammatory Cytokines Within the Central Nervous System: Sources, Function, and Mechanism of Action," *American Journal of Physiology* 263, no. 1, pt. 1 (1992): C1–C16; S. F. Maier, L. E. Goehler, M. Fleshner, et al., "The Role of the Vagus Nerve in Cytokine-to-Brain Communication," *Annals of the New York Academy of Sciences* (1998), doi: 10.1111/j.1749-6632.1998.tb09569.x.

52. F. Belardelli and M. Ferrantini, "Cytokines as a Link Between Innate and Adaptive Antitumor Immunity," *Trends in Immunology* 23, no. 4 (2002): 201–208, doi: 10.1016/S1471-4906(02)02195-6; A. Iwasaki and R. Medzhitov, "Control of Adaptive Immunity by the Innate Immune System," *Nature Immunology* 16, no. 4 (2015): 343–353, doi: 10.1038/ni.3123.

53. A. Qaseem, T. J. Wilt, R. M. McLean, et al., "Noninvasive Treatments for Acute, Subacute, and Chronic Low Back Pain: A Clinical Practice Guideline from the American College of Physicians," *Annals of Internal Medicine* 166, no. 7 (2017): 514–530, doi: 10.7326/M16-2367.

Chapter 7: Can We Heal Each Other? Biofield Therapies and Health

1. M. Hofman, J. L. Ryan, C. D. Figueroa-Moseley, et al., "Cancer-Related Fatigue: The Scale of the Problem," *Oncologist* 12, no. S1 (2007): 4–10, doi: 10.1634/theoncologist.12-S1-4.

2. J. E. Bower, "Cancer-Related Fatigue: Mechanisms, Risk Factors, and Treatments," *Nature Reviews Clinical Oncology* 11, no. 10 (2014): 597.

3. R. Bruyere, *Wheels of Light: Chakras, Auras, and the Healing Energy of the Body* (New York: Simon and Schuster, 1994).

4. I. Golden, "Beyond Randomized Controlled Trials: Evidence in Complementary Medicine," *Evidence-Based Complementary and Alternative Medicine* 17, no. 1 (2012): 72–75, doi: 10.1177/2156587211429351.

5. S. Jain, D. Pavlik, J. Distefan, et al., "Complementary Medicine for Fatigue and Cortisol Variability in Breast Cancer Survivors: A Randomized Controlled Trial," *Cancer* 118, no. 3 (2012): 777–787, doi: 10.1002/cncr.26345.

6. N. Petrovsky, P. McNair, and L. C. Harrison, "Diurnal Rhythms of Pro-Inflammatory Cytokines: Regulation by Plasma Cortisol and Therapeutic Implications," *Cytokine* 10, no. 4 (1998): 307–312, doi: 10.1006/cyto.1997.0289.

7. S. E. Sephton, R. M. Sapolsky, H. C. Kraemer, et al., "Diurnal Cortisol Rhythm as a Predictor of Breast Cancer Survival," *Journal of the National Cancer Institute* 92, no. 12 (2000): 994–1000.

8. M. H. Antoni, S. K. Lutgendorf, S. W. Cole, et al., "The Influence of Bio-Behavioural Factors on Tumour Biology: Pathways and Mechanisms," *Nature Reviews Cancer* 6, no. 3 (2006): 240–248, doi: 10.1038/nrc1820.

9. S. K. Lutgendorf, E. Mullen-Houser, D. Russell, et al., "Preservation of Immune Function in Cervical Cancer Patients During Chemoradiation Using a Novel Integrative Approach," *Brain, Behavior, and Immunity* 24, no. 8 (2010): 1231–1240, doi: 10.1016/j.bbi.2010.06.014.

10. S. Jain and P. J. Mills, "Biofield Therapies: Helpful or Full of Hype? A Best Evidence Synthesis," *International Journal of Complementary Medicine* 17 (2010), doi: 10.1007/s12529-009-9062-4.

11. P. S. So, Y. Jiang, and Y. Qin, "Touch Therapies for Pain Relief in Adults," *Cochrane Database of Systematic Reviews* (2008), doi: 10.1002/14651858.CD006535.pub2.

12. M. Demir Doğan, "The Effect of Reiki on Pain: A Meta-Analysis," *Complementary Therapies in Clinical Practice* 31 (2018): 384–387, doi: 10.1016/j.ctcp.2018.02.020.

13. A. Bardia, D. L. Barton, L. J. Prokop, et al., "Efficacy of Complementary and Alternative Medicine Therapies in Relieving Cancer Pain: A Systematic Review," *Journal of Clinical Oncology* 24, no. 34 (2006): 5457–5464, doi: 10.1200/JCO.2006.08.3725.

14. J. Joyce and G. P. Herbison, "Reiki for Depression and Anxiety," *Cochrane Database of Systematic Reviews* 4 (2015): CD006833, doi: 10.1002/14651858.CD006833.pub2.

15. J. A. Maville, J. E. Bowen, and G. Benham, "Effect of Healing Touch on Stress Perception and Biological Correlates," *Holistic Nursing Practice* 22, no. 2 (2008): 103–110.

16. D. S. Wilkinson, P. L. Knox, J. E. Chatman, et al., "The Clinical Effectiveness of Healing Touch," *Journal of Alternative and Complementary Medicine* 8, no. 1 (2002): 33–47; L. Díaz-Rodríguez, M. Arroyo-Morales, I. Cantarero-Villanueva, et al., "The Application of Reiki in Nurses Diagnosed with Burnout Syndrome Has Beneficial Effects on Concentration of Salivary IgA and Blood Pressure," *Revista Latino-Americana de Enfermagem* 19, no. 5 (2011): 1132–1138, doi: 10.1590/S0104-11692011000500010; R. S. Friedman, M. M. Burg, P. Miles, et al., "Effects of Reiki on Autonomic Activity Early after Acute Coronary Syndrome," *Journal of the American College of Cardiology* 56, no. 12 (2010): 995–996; D. W. Wardell and J. Engebretson, "Biological Correlates of Reiki Touch(sm) Healing," *Journal of Advanced Nursing* 33, no. 4 (2001): 439–445, doi: 10.1046/j.1365-2648.2001.01691.x; J. Achterberg, K. Cooke, T. Richards, et al., "Evidence for Correlations Between Distant Intentionality and Brain Function in Recipients: A Functional Magnetic Resonance Imaging Analysis," *Journal of Alternative and Complementary Medicine* 11, no. 6 (2005): 965–971, doi: 10.1089/acm.2005.11.965.

17. Hammerschlag R, Marx BL, and Aickin M, "Nontouch Biofield Therapy: A Systematic Review of Human Randomized Controlled Trials Reporting Use of Only Nonphysical Contact Treatment," *Journal of Alternative and Complementary Medicine* 20, no. 12 (2014): 881–92, doi: 10.1089/acm.2014.0017.

18. Association for Comprehensive Energy Psychology (ACEP), *What Is Energy Psychology?* (Bryn Mawr, PA: ACEP, 2020), cdn.ymaws.com/www.energypsych.org/resource/resmgr/What_is_Energy_Psychology_20.pdf.

19. M. Clond, "Emotional Freedom Techniques for Anxiety: A Systematic Review with Meta-Analysis," *Journal of Nervous and Mental Disease* 204, no. 5 (2016): 388–395, doi: 10.1097/NMD.0000000000000483.

20. J. A. Nelms and L. Castel, "A Systematic Review and Meta-Analysis of Randomized and Nonrandomized Trials of Clinical Emotional Freedom Techniques (EFT) for the Treatment of Depression," *Explore* 12, no. 6 (2016): 416–426, doi: 10.1016/j.explore.2016.08.001.

21. B. Sebastian and J. Nelms, "The Effectiveness of Emotional Freedom Techniques in the Treatment of Posttraumatic Stress Disorder: A Meta-Analysis," *Explore* 13, no. 1 (2017): 16–25, doi: 10.1016/j.explore.2016.10.001.

22. D. Church, G. Yount, K. Rachlin, et al., "Epigenetic Effects of PTSD Remediation in Veterans Using Clinical Emotional Freedom Techniques: A Randomized Controlled Pilot Study," *American Journal of Health Promotion* 32, no. 1 (2018): 112–122, doi: 10.1177/0890117116661154.

23. D. Radin, M. Schlitz, and C. Baur, "Distant Healing Intention Therapies: An Overview of the Scientific Evidence," *Global Advances in Health and Medicine* 4, Suppl. (2015): doi: 10.7453/gahmj.2015.012.suppl.

24. S. Schmidt, R. Schneider, J. Utts, et al., "Distant Intentionality and the Feeling of Being Stared At: Two Meta-Analyses," *British Journal of Psychology* 95, pt. 2 (2004): 235–247, doi: 10.1348/000712604773952449.

25. C. A. Roe, C. Sonnex, and E. C. Roxburgh, "Two Meta-Analyses of Noncontact Healing Studies," *Explore* 11, no. 1 (2015): 11–23, doi: 10.1016/j.explore.2014 .10.001.

26. J. A. Astin, E. Harkness, and E. Ernst, "The Efficacy of 'Distant Healing': A Systematic Review of Randomized Trials," *Annals of Internal Medicine* 132, no. 11 (2000): 903–910, doi: 10.7326/0003-4819-132-11-200006060-00009.

27. E. Ernst, "Distant Healing: An 'Update' of a Systematic Review," *Wiener Klinische Wochenschrift* 115, nos. 7–8 (2003): 241–245, doi: 10.1007/BF03040322.

28. W. B. Jonas, "The Middle Way: Realistic Randomized Controlled Trials for the Evaluation of Spiritual Healing," *Journal of Alternative and Complementary Medicine* 7, no. 1 (2001): 5–7, doi: 10.1089/107555301300004466.

29. L. Roberts, I. Ahmed, and A. Davison, "Intercessory Prayer for the Alleviation of Ill Health," *Cochrane Database of Systematic Reviews* 2009, no. 2 (2009), doi: 10.1002/14651858.CD000368.pub3.

30. K. S. Masters, G. I. Spielmans, and J. T. Goodson, "Are There Demonstrable Effects of Distant Intercessory Prayer? A Meta-Analytic Review," *Annals of Behavioral Medicine* 32, no. 1 (2006): 21–26, doi: 10.1207/s15324796abm3201_3.

31. J. Engebretson and D. W. Wardell, "Energy Therapies: Focus on Spirituality," *Explore* 8, no. 6 (2012): 353–359, doi: 10.1016/j.explore.2012.08.004; J. Engebretson and D. W. Wardell, "Experience of a Reiki Session," *Alternative Therapies in Health and Medicine* 8, no. 2 (2002): 48–53; B. M. H. Stöckigt, F. Besch, F. Jeserich, et al., "Healing Relationships: A Qualitative Study of Healers and Their Clients in Germany," *Evidence-Based Complementary and Alternative Medicine*, doi: 10.1155/2015/145154.

Chapter 8: Healing Down to Our Cells

1. I. Kalajzic, Z. Kalajzic, M. Kaliterna, et al., "Use of Type I Collagen Green Fluorescent Protein Transgenes to Identify Subpopulations of Cells at Different Stages of the Osteoblast Lineage," *Journal of Bone and Mineral Research* 17, no. 1 (2002): 15–25, doi: 10.1359/jbmr.2002.17.1.15; S. Sofia, M. B. McCarthy, G. Gronowicz, et al., "Functionalized Silk-Based Biomaterials for Bone Formation,"

Journal of Biomedical Materials Reseach 54, no. 1 (2001): 139–148, doi: 10.1002/1097-4636(200101)54:1<139::aid-jbm17>3.0.co;2-7.

2. G. A. Gronowicz, A. Jhaveri, L. W. Clarke, et al., "Therapeutic Touch Stimulates the Proliferation of Human Cells in Culture," *Journal of Alternative and Complementary Medicine* 14, no. 3 (2008): 233–239, doi: 10.1089/acm.2007.7163.

3. A. Jhaveri, S. J. Walsh, Y. Wang, et al., "Therapeutic Touch Affects DNA Synthesis and Mineralization of Human Osteoblasts in Culture," *Journal of Orthopaedic Research* 26, no. 11 (2008): 1541–1546, doi: 10.1002/jor.20688.

4. X. Yan, H. Shen, H. Jiang, et al., "External Qi of Yan Xin Qigong Differentially Regulates the Akt and Extracellular Signal-Regulated Kinase Pathways and Is Cytotoxic to Cancer Cells but Not to Normal Cells," *International Journal of Biochemistry and Cell Biology* 38, no. 12 (2006): 2102–2113, doi: 10.1016 /j.biocel.2006.06.002.

5. A. Arlt, A. Gehrz, S. Müerköster, et al., "Role of NF-kappaB and Akt/PI3K in the Resistance of Pancreatic Carcinoma Cell Lines Against Gemcitabine-Induced Cell Death," *Oncogene* 22, no. 21 (2003): 3243–3251, doi: 10.1038/sj.onc.1206390; T. Asano, Y. Yao, J. Zhu, et al., "The PI 3-kinase/Akt Signaling Pathway Is Activated Due to Aberrant Pten Expression and Targets Transcription Factors NF-kappaB and c-Myc in Pancreatic Cancer Cells," *Oncogene* 23, no. 53 (2004): 8571–8580, doi: 10.1038/sj.onc.1207902.

6. V. Asati, D. K. Mahapatra, and S. K. Bharti, "PI 3K/Akt/mTOR and Ras/Raf/ MEK/ERK Signaling Pathways Inhibitors as Anticancer Agents: Structural and Pharmacological Perspectives," *European Journal of Medicinal Chemistry* 109 (2016): 314–341, doi: 10.1016/j.ejmech.2016.01.012.

7. X. Yan, H. Shen, H. Jiang, et al., "External Qi of Yan Xin Qigong Induces Apoptosis and Inhibits Migration and Invasion of Estrogen-Independent Breast Cancer Cells Through Suppression of Akt/NF-\KB Signaling," *Cellular Physiology and Biochemistry* 25, nos. 2–3 (2010): 263–270; X. Yan, H. Shen, H. Jiang, et al., "External Qi of Yan Xin Qigong Inhibits Activation of Akt, Erk1/2, and NF-\KB and Induces Cell Cycle Arrest and Apoptosis in Colorectal Cancer Cells," *Cellular Physiology and Biochemistry* 31, no. 1 (2013): 113–122; X. Yan, H. Shen, H. Jiang, et al., "External Qi of Yan Xin Qigong Induces G2/M Arrest and Apoptosis of Androgen-Independent Prostate Cancer Cells by Inhibiting Akt and NF-xB Pathways," *Molecular and Cellular Biochemistry* 310, nos. 1–2 (2008): 227–234.

8. G. Gronowicz, E. R. Secor, J. R. Flynn, et al., "Therapeutic Touch Has Significant Effects on Mouse Breast Cancer Metastasis and Immune Responses but Not Primary Tumor Size," *Evidence-Based Complementary and Alternative Medicine* (2015): 926565, doi: 10.1155/2015/926565.

9. W. F. Bengston and D. Krinsley, "The Effect of the 'Laying on of Hands' on Transplanted Breast Cancer in Mice," *Journal of Scientific Explorarion* 14, no. 3 (2000): 353–364; W. F. Bengston, "Spirituality, Connection, and Healing with

Intent: Reflections on Cancer Experiments on Laboratory Mice," in *The Oxford Handbook of Psychology and Spirituality* (Oxford, UK: Oxford University Press, 2012), 548–557, doi: 10.1093/oxfordhb/9780199729920.013.0035.

10. W. Bengston, *The Energy Cure: Unraveling the Mystery of Hands-on Healing* (Boulder, CO: Sounds True, 2010).

11. W. Bengston, "Examining Biological and Physical Correlates to Anomalous Healing," *Journal of the American Holistic Veterinary Medical Association* 55 (2019).

12. M. M. Moga and W. F. Bengston, "Anomalous Magnetic Field Activity During a Bioenergy Healing Experiment," *Journal of Scientific Exploration* 24, no. 3 (2010): 397–410.

13. M. M. Karbowski, S. L. Harribance, C. A. Buckner, et al., "Digitized Quantitative Electroencephalographic Patterns Applied as Magnetic Fields Inhibit Melanoma Cell Proliferation in Culture," *Neuroscience Letters* 523, no. 2 (2012): 131–134; M. A. Persinger and K. S. Saroka, "Protracted Parahippocampal Activity Associated with Sean Harribance," *International Journal of Yoga* 5, no. 2 (2012): 140; W. G. Roll and M. A. Persinger, "Is ESP a Form of Perception? Contributions from a Study of Sean Harribance," *Journal of Parapsychology* 62, no. 2 (1998): 117.

14. P. Yang, Y. Jiang, P. R. Rhea, et al., "Human Biofield Therapy and the Growth of Mouse Lung Carcinoma," *Integrative Cancer Therapies* 18 (2019): doi: 10.1177/1534735419840797.

15. L. Wilson, "Effects of Environmental Stress on the Architecture and Permeability of the Rat Mesenteric Microvasculature," *Microcirculation* 5 (1998): 299–308, doi: 10.1111/j.1549-8719.1998.tb00079.x; M. Jain and A. L. Baldwin, "Are Laboratory Animals Stressed by Their Housing Environment and Are Investigators Aware That This Stress Can Affect Physiological Data?" *Medical Hypotheses* 60, no. 2 (2003): 284–289, doi: 10.1016/s0306-9877(02)00387-0.

16. A. L. Baldwin and G. E. Schwartz, "Personal Interaction with a Reiki Practitioner Decreases Noise-Induced Microvascular Damage in an Animal Model," *Journal of Alternative and Complementary Medicine* 12, no. 1 (2006): 15–22, doi: 10.1089/acm.2006.12.15.

17. A. L. Baldwin, C. Wagers, and G. E. Schwartz, "Reiki Improves Heart Rate Homeostasis in Laboratory Rats," *Journal of Alternative and Complementary Medicine* 14, no. 4 (2008): 417–422, doi: 10.1089/acm.2007.0753; A. L. Baldwin, W. L. Rand, and G. E. Schwartz, "Practicing Reiki Does Not Appear to Routinely Produce High-Intensity Electromagnetic Fields from the Heart or Hands of Reiki Practitioners," *Journal of Alternative and Complementary Medicine* 19, no. 6 (2012): 518–526, doi: 10.1089/acm.2012.0136; A. L. Baldwin, A. Vitale, E. Brownell, et al., "Effects of Reiki on Pain, Anxiety, and Blood Pressure in Patients Undergoing Knee Replacement: A Pilot Study," *Holistic Nursing Practice* 31, no. 2 (2017): 80–89, doi: 10.1097/HNP.0000000000000195.

18. M. M. Moga and D. Zhou, "Distant Healing of Small-Sized Tumors," *Journal of Alternative and Complementary Medicine* 14, no. 5 (2008): 453, doi: 10.1089

/acm.2008.0100; X. Yan, F. Li, I. Dozmorov, et al., "External Qi of Yan Xin Qigong Induces Cell Death and Gene Expression Alterations Promoting Apoptosis and Inhibiting Proliferation, Migration, and Glucose Metabolism in Small-Cell Lung Cancer Cells," *Molecular and Cellular Biochemistry* 363, nos. 1–2 (2012): 245–255.

19. R. Hammerschlag, S. Jain, A. L. Baldwin, et al., "Biofield Research: A Roundtable Discussion of Scientific and Methodological Issues," *Journal of Alternative and Complementary Medicine* 18, no. 12 (2012): 1081–1086, doi: 10.1089/acm.2012.1502.

20. G. Gronowicz, W. Bengston, and G. Yount, "Challenges for Preclinical Investigations of Human Biofield Modalities," *Global Advances in Health and Medicine* 4, Suppl. (2015): 52–57; J. G. Kiang, J. A. Ives, and W. B. Jonas, "External Bioenergy-Induced Increases in Intracellular Free Calcium Concentrations Are Mediated by Na+/Ca2+ Exchanger and L-Type Calcium Channel," *Molecular and Cellular Biochemistry* 271, nos. 1–2 (2005): 51–59, doi: 10.1007/s11010-005-3615-x.

21. G. Yount, J. Solfvin, D. Moore, et al., "In Vitro Test of External Qigong," *BMC Complementary and Alternative Medicine* 4 (2004): 5, doi: 10.1186/1472-6882-4-5.

Chapter 9: What's the "Mechanism" for Biofield Healing?

1. K. J. Kemper and H. A. Shaltout, "Non-Verbal Communication of Compassion: Measuring Psychophysiologic Effects," *BMC Complementary and Alternative Medicine* 11 (2011): 132, doi: 10.1186/1472-6882-11-132.

2. D. Tilliman, "The Effects of Unconditional Positive Regard on Psychotherapy Outcome," *Dissertation Abstracts International* 77, no. 10-B(E) (2017); P. Wilkins, "Unconditional Positive Regard Reconsidered," *British Journal of Guidance and Counselling* 28, no. 1 (2000): 23–36, doi: 10.1080/030698800109592.

3. R. H. W. Funk, T. Monsees, and N. Ozkucur, "Electromagnetic Effects: From Cell Biology to Medicine," *Progress in Histochemistry and Cytochemistry* 43, no. 4 (2009): 177–264, doi: 10.1016/j.proghi.2008.07.001.

4. J. A. Ives, E. P. A. Van Wijk, N. Bat, et al., "Ultraweak Photon Emission as a Non-Invasive Health Assessment: A Systematic Review," *PLoS One* 9, no. 2 (2014): e87401, doi: 10.1371/journal.pone.0087401.

5. R. Hammerschlag, M. Levin, R. McCraty, et al., "Biofield Physiology: A Framework for an Emerging Discipline," *Global Advances in Health and Medicine* 4, Suppl. (2015).

6. B. Rubik, "Measurement of the Human Biofield and Other Energetic Instruments," *Mosby's Complementary and Alternative Medicine: A Research-Based Approach* (Maryland Heights, MO: Mosby, 2009): 555–573.

7. M. A. Persinger and K. S. Saroka, "Protracted Parahippocampal Activity Associated with Sean Harribance," *International Journal of Yoga* 5, no. 2 (2012): 140; M. A. Persinger, "The Harribance Effect as Pervasive Out-of-Body Experiences: NeuroQuantal Evidence with More Precise Measurements," *NeuroQuantology* 8, no. 4 (2010); A. Seto, C. Kusaka, S. Nakazato, et al., "Detection of Extraordinary Large Bio-Magnetic Field Strength from Human Hand During External Qi

Emission," *Acupuncture and Electro-Therapeutics Research* 17, no. 2 (1992): 75–94, doi: 10.3727/036012992816357819; T. Hisamitsu, A. Seto, S. Nakazato, et al., "Emission of Extremely Strong Magnetic Fields from the Head and Whole Body During Oriental Breathing Exercises," *Acupuncture and Electro-Therapeutics Research* 21, nos. 3–4 (1996): 219–227, doi: 10.3727/036012996816356898; B. Rubik and H. Jabs, "Effects of Intention, Energy Healing, and Mind-Body States on Biophoton Emission," *Cosmos and History: The Journal of Natural and Social Philosophy* 13, no. 2 (2017): 227–247; K. W. Chen, "An Analytic Review of Studies on Measuring Effects of External Qi in China," *Alternative Therapies in Health and Medicine* 10, no. 4 (2004): 38–51.

8. A. L. Baldwin, W. L. Rand, and G. E. Schwartz, "Practicing Reiki Does Not Appear to Routinely Produce High-Intensity Electromagnetic Fields from the Heart or Hands of Reiki Practitioners," *Journal of Alternative and Complementary Medicine* 19, no. 6 (2012): 518–526, doi: 10.1089/acm.2012.0136.

9. I. Tatarov, A. Panda, D. Petkov, et al., "Effect of Magnetic Fields on Tumor Growth and Viability," *Comparative Medicine* 61, no. 4 (2011): 339–345; S. Crocetti, C. Beyer, G. Schade, et al., "Low Intensity and Frequency Pulsed Electromagnetic Fields Selectively Impair Breast Cancer Cell Viability," *PLoS One* 8, no. 9 (2013): e72944, doi: 10.1371/journal.pone.0072944; J. Rick, A. Chandra, and M. K. Aghi, "Tumor Treating Fields: A New Approach to Glioblastoma Therapy," *Journal of Neuro-Oncology* 137, no. 3 (2018): 447–453, doi: 10.1007/s11060-018-2768-x; R. Stupp, S. Taillibert, A. Kanner, et al., "Effect of Tumor-Treating Fields Plus Maintenance Temozolomide vs. Maintenance Temozolomide Alone on Survival in Patients with Glioblastoma: A Randomized Clinical Trial," *JAMA* 318, no. 23 (2017): 2306–2316, doi: 10.1001/jama.2017.18718; C. L. Ross, M. Siriwardane, G. Almeida-Porada, et al., "The Effect of Low-Frequency Electromagnetic Field on Human Bone Marrow Stem/Progenitor Cell Differentiation," *Stem Cell Research* 15, no. 1 (2015): 96–108, doi: 10.1016/j.scr.2015.04.009; X. L. Griffin, M. L. Costa, N. Parsons, et al., "Electromagnetic Field Stimulation for Treating Delayed Union or Non-Union of Long Bone Fractures in Adults," *Cochrane Database of Systematic Reviews* 4 (2011): CD008471, doi: 10.1002/14651858.CD008471.pub2; B. Zhang, Y. Xie, Z. Ni, et al., "Effects and Mechanisms of Exogenous Electromagnetic Field on Bone Cells: A Review," *Bioelectromagnetics* 41, no. 4 (2020): 263–278, doi: 10.1002/bem.22258.

10. H. Lin, M. Blank, K. Rossol-Haseroth, et al., "Regulating Genes with Electromagnetic Response Elements," *Journal of Cellular Biochemistry* 81, no. 1 (2001): 143–148, doi: 10.1002/1097-4644(20010401)81:1<143::aid-jcb1030>3.0.co;2-4; A. O. Rodríguez de la Fuente, J. M. Alcocer-González, J. Antonio Heredia-Rojas, et al., "Effect of 60 Hz Electromagnetic Fields on the Activity of hsp70 Promoter: An in Vitro Study," *Cell Biology International* 33, no. 3 (2009): 419–423, doi: 10.1016/j.cellbi.2008.09.014.

11. M. Blank and R. Goodman, "Electromagnetic Initiation of Transcription at Specific DNA Sites," *Journal of Cellular Biochemistry* 81, no. 4 (2001): 689–692, doi: 10.1002/jcb.1102.

12. M. L. Pall, "Electromagnetic Fields Act via Activation of Voltage-Gated Calcium Channels to Produce Beneficial or Adverse Effects," *Journal of Cellular and Molecular Medicine* 17, no. 8 (2013): 958–965, doi: 10.1111/jcmm.12088.

13. J. G. Kiang, J. A. Ives, and W. B. Jonas, "External Bioenergy-Induced Increases in Intracellular Free Calcium Concentrations Are Mediated by Na+/Ca2+ Exchanger and L-Type Calcium Channel," *Molecular and Cellular Biochemistry* 271, nos. 1–2 (2005): 51–59, doi: 10.1007/s11010-005-3615-x.

14. P. C. Benias, R. G. Wells, B. Sackey-Aboagye, et al., "Structure and Distribution of an Unrecognized Interstitium in Human Tissues," *Scientific Reports* 8, no. 1 (2018): 4947, doi: 10.1038/s41598-018-23062-6.

15. H. M. Langevin and J. A. Yandow, "Relationship of Acupuncture Points and Meridians to Connective Tissue Planes," *Anatomical Record* 269, no. 6 (2002): 257–265, doi: 10.1002/ar.10185.

16. A. C. Ahn, J. Wu, G. J. Badger, et al., "Electrical Impedance along Connective Tissue Planes Associated with Acupuncture Meridians," *BMC Complementary and Alternative Medicine* 5 (2005): 10, doi: 10.1186/1472-6882-5-10; A. C. Ahn, M. Park, J. R. Shaw, et al., "Electrical Impedance of Acupuncture Meridians: The Relevance of Subcutaneous Collagenous Bands," *PLoS One* 5, no. 7 (2010): e11907, doi: 10.1371/journal.pone.0011907; A. C. Ahn, A. P. Colbert, B. J. Anderson, et al., "Electrical Properties of Acupuncture Points and Meridians: A Systematic Review," *Bioelectromagnetics* 29, no. 4 (2008): 245–256, doi: 10.1002/bem.20403.

17. M.-W. Ho and D. P. Knight, "The Acupuncture System and the Liquid Crystalline Collagen Fibers of the Connective Tissues," *American Journal of Chinese Medicine* 26, nos. 3–4 (1998): 251–263, doi: 10.1142/S0192415X98000294; M.-W. Ho, *The Rainbow and the Worm: The Physics of Organisms* (Singapore: World Scientific, 2008).

18. J. L. Oschman, *Energy Medicine: The Scientific Basis* (New York: Elsevier Health Sciences, 2015).

19. K. Heaney, "Do We Finally Understand How Acupuncture Works?" *The Cut*, March 30, 2018, thecut.com/2018/03/do-we-finally-understand-how-acupuncture-works.html.

20. R. A. Briggaman and C. E. Wheeler, "The Epidermal-Dermal Junction," *Journal of Investigative Dermatology* 65, no. 1 (1975): 71–84, doi: 10.1111/1523-1747.ep12598050.

21. J. Abraham and S. Mathew, "Merkel Cells: A Collective Review of Current Concepts," *International Journal of Applied and Basic Medical Research* 9, no. 1 (2019): 9–13, doi: 10.4103/ijabmr.IJABMR_34_18; S. Maksimovic, M. Nakatani, Y. Baba, et al., "Epidermal Merkel Cells Are Mechanosensory Cells That Tune Mammalian Touch Receptors," *Nature* 509, no. 7502 (2014): 617–621, doi: 10.1038/nature13250;

K. M. Morrison, G. R. Miesegaes, E. A. Lumpkin, et al., "Mammalian Merkel Cells Are Descended from the Epidermal Lineage," *Developmental Biology* 336, no. 1 (2009): 76–83, doi: 10.1016/j.ydbio.2009.09.032; M. K. Irmak, E. Oztas, M. Yagmurca, et al., "Effects of Electromagnetic Radiation from a Cellular Telephone on Epidermal Merkel Cells," *Journal of Cutaneous Pathology* 30 (2003): 135–138, doi: 10.1046/j.0303-6987.2003.00002.x; S.-H. Woo, S. Ranade, A. D. Weyer, et al., "Piezo2 Is Required for Merkel-Cell Mechanotransduction," *Nature* 509, no. 7502 (2014): 622–626, doi: 10.1038/nature13251.

22. B. U. Hoffman, Y. Baba, T. N. Griffith, et al., "Merkel Cells Activate Sensory Neural Pathways Through Adrenergic Synapses," *Neuron* 100, no. 6 (2018): 1401–1413, doi: 10.1016/j.neuron.2018.10.034.

23. M. K. Irmak, "Multifunctional Merkel Cells: Their Roles in Electromagnetic Reception, Finger-Print Formation, Reiki, Epigenetic Inheritance, and Hair Form," *Medical Hypotheses* 75, no. 2 (2010): 162–168, doi: 10.1016/j.mehy.2010.02.011.

24. B. Julsgaard, A. Kozhekin, and E. S. Polzik, "Experimental Long-Lived Entanglement of Two Macroscopic Objects," *Nature* 413, no. 6854 (2001): 400–403, doi: 10.1038/35096524; P. Zarkeshian, C. Deshmukh, N. Sinclair, et al., "Entanglement Between More Than Two Hundred Macroscopic Atomic Ensembles in a Solid," *Nature Communications* 8, no. 1 (2017): 906, doi: 10.1038/s41467-017-00897-7; A. Bulgac and S. Jin, "Dynamics of Fragmented Condensates and Macroscopic Entanglement," *Physical Review Letters* 119, no. 5 (2017): 052501, doi: 10.1103/PhysRevLett.119.052501; C.-S. Hu, X.-Y. Lin, L.-T. Shen, et al., "Improving Macroscopic Entanglement with Nonlocal Mechanical Squeezing," *Optics Express* 28, no. 2 (2020): 1492–1506, doi: 10.1364/OE.379058; X. Huang, E. Zeuthen, D. V. Vasilyev, et al., "Unconditional Steady-State Entanglement in Macroscopic Hybrid Systems by Coherent Noise Cancellation," *Physical Review Letters* 121, no. 10 (2018): 103602, doi: 10.1103/PhysRevLett.121.103602; K. C. Lee, M. R. Sprague, B. J. Sussman, et al., "Entangling Macroscopic Diamonds at Room Temperature," *Science* 334, no. 6060 (2011): 1253–1256, doi: 10.1126/science.1211914.

25. A. Furusawa, J. L. Sorensen, S. L. Braunstein, et al., "Unconditional Quantum Teleportation," *Science* 282, no. 5389 (1998): 706–709, doi: 10.1126/science.282.5389.706; W. Pfaff, B. J. Hensen, H. Bernien, et al., "Quantum Information: Unconditional Quantum Teleportation Between Distant Solid-State Quantum Bits," *Science* 345, no. 6196 (2014): 532–535, doi: 10.1126/science.1253512.

26. J.-G. Ren, P. Xu, H.-L. Yong, et al., "Ground-to-Satellite Quantum Teleportation," *Nature* 549, no. 7670 (2017): 70–73, doi: 10.1038/nature23675.

27. J. McFadden and J. al-Khalili, "The Origins of Quantum Biology," *Proceedings of the Royal Society A: Mathematical, Physical and Engineering Sciences* 474, no. 2220 (2018): 20180674, doi: 10.1098/rspa.2018.0674; J. Zhu, S. Kais, A. Aspuru-Guzik, et al., "Multipartite Quantum Entanglement Evolution in Photosynthetic Complexes," *Journal of Chemical Physics* 137, no. 7 (2012): 074112, doi: 10.1063/1.4742333; J. C. Brookes, "Quantum Effects in Biology: Golden Rule

in Enzymes, Olfaction, Photosynthesis, and Magnetodetection," *Proceedings: Mathematical, Physical, and Engineering Sciences* 473, no. 2201 (2017): 20160822, doi: 10.1098/rspa.2016.0822; A. Tamulis and M. Grigalavicius, "Quantum Entanglement in Photoactive Prebiotic Systems," *Systems and Synthetic Biology* 8, no. 2 (2014): 117–140, doi: 10.1007/s11693-014-9138-6.

28. H. Stuart, "Quantum Computation in Brain Microtubules? The Penrose-Hameroff 'Orch OR' Model of Consciousness," *Philosophical Transactions of the Royal Society of London Series A: Mathematical, Physical, and Engineering Sciences* 356, no. 1743 (1998): 1869–1896; S. Hameroff and R. Penrose, "Consciousness in the Universe: A Review of the 'Orch OR' Theory," *Physics of Life Reviews* 11, no. 1 (2014): 39–78.

29. H. J. Hogben, T. Biskup, and P. J. Hore, "Entanglement and Sources of Magnetic Anisotropy in Radical Pair-Based Avian Magnetoreceptors," *Physical Review Letters* 109, no. 22 (2012): 220501, doi: 10.1103/PhysRevLett.109.220501; E. M. Gauger, E. Rieper, J. J. L. Morton, et al., "Sustained Quantum Coherence and Entanglement in the Avian Compass," *Physical Review Letters* 106, no. 4 (2011): 040503, doi: 10.1103/PhysRevLett.106.040503; J. A. Pauls, Y. Zhang, G. P. Berman, et al., "Quantum Coherence and Entanglement in the Avian Compass," *Physical Review E: Statistical, Nonlinear, and Soft Matter Physics* 87, no. 6 (2013): 062704, doi: 10.1103/PhysRevE.87.062704.

30. C. Mothersill, R. Smith, J. Wang, et al., "Biological Entanglement–Like Effect after Communication of Fish Prior to X-Ray Exposure," *Dose Response* 16, no. 1 (2018): 1559325817750067, doi: 10.1177/1559325817750067.

31. G. Zukav, *The Dancing Wu Li Masters: An Overview of the New Physics* (New York: Random House, 2012); H. P. Stapp. "Mind, Matter, and Quantum Mechanics," *Foundations of Physics* 12, no. 4 (1982): 363–399; M. C. Kafatos and K.-H. Yang, "The Quantum Universe: Philosophical Foundations and Oriental Medicine," *Integrative Medicine Research* 5, no. 4 (2016): 237–243, doi: 10.1016 /j.imr.2016.08.003; M. Kafatos and R. Nadeau, *The Conscious Universe: Part and Whole in Modern Physical Theory* (New York: Springer, 2012).

32. M. C. Kafatos, G. Chevalier, D. Chopra, et al., "Biofield Science: Current Physics Perspectives," *Global Advances in Health and Medicine* 4, Suppl. (2015): doi: 10.7453/gahmj.2015.011.suppl.

33. Y. Li, A. Nemilentsau, and C. Argyropoulos, "Resonance Energy Transfer and Quantum Entanglement Mediated by Epsilon-Near-Zero and Other Plasmonic Waveguide Systems," *Nanoscale* 11, no. 31 (2019): 14635–14647, doi: 10.1039 /c9nr05083c; K. Najafi, A. L. Wysocki, K. Park, et al., "Toward Long-Range Entanglement Between Electrically Driven Single-Molecule Magnets," *Journal of Physical Chemistry Letters* 10, no. 23 (2019): 7347–7355, doi: 10.1021 /acs.jpclett.9b03131.

34. E. Megidish, A. Halevy, T. Shacham, et al., "Entanglement Swapping Between Photons That Have Never Coexisted," *Physical Review Letters* 110, no. 21 (2013): 210403, doi: 10.1103/PhysRevLett.110.210403.

35. E. A. Sobie, S. Guatimosim, L.-S. Song, et al., "The Challenge of Molecular Medicine: Complexity Versus Occam's Razor," *Journal of Clinical Investigations* 111, no. 6 (2003): 801–803, doi: 10.1172/JCI18153.

36. L. Carpenter, H. Wahbeh, G. Yount, et al., "Possible Negentropic Effects Observed During Energy Medicine Sessions," *Explore* 17, no. 1 (2021): 45–49; G. Yount, A. Delorme, D. Radin, et al., "Energy Medicine Treatments for Hand and Wrist Pain: A Pilot Study," *Explore* 17, no. 1 (2021): 11–21.

37. H. Wahbeh, E. Niebauer, A. Delorme, et al., "A Case Study of Extended Human Capacity Perception During Energy Medicine Treatments Using Mixed Methods Analysis," *Explore* 17, no. 1 (2021): 70–78.

Chapter 10: Ground for Health

1. E. Fukada and I. Yasuda, "On the Piezoelectric Effect of Bone," *Journal of the Physical Society of Japan* (1957), doi: 10.1143/JPSJ.12.1158; J. A. Ives, E. P. A. Van Wijk, N. Bat, et al., "Ultraweak Photon Emission as a Non-Invasive Health Assessment: A Systematic Review," *PLoS One* 9, no. 2 (2014), doi: 10.1371/journal.pone.0087401.

2. C. X. Wang, I. A. Hilburn, D. A. Wu, et al., "Transduction of the Geomagnetic Field as Evidenced from Alpha-Band Activity in the Human Brain," *eNeuro* (2019), doi: 10.1523/ENEURO.0483-18.2019; A. Alabdulgader, R. McCraty, M. Atkinson, et al., "Long-Term Study of Heart Rate Variability Responses to Changes in the Solar and Geomagnetic Environment," *Scientific Reports* (2018), doi: 10.1038/s41598-018-20932-x; V. A. Ozheredov, S. M. Chibisov, M. L. Blagonravov, et al., "Influence of Geomagnetic Activity and Earth Weather Changes on Heart Rate and Blood Pressure in Young and Healthy Population," *International Journal of Biometeorology* (2017), doi: 10.1007/s00484-016-1272-2.

3. J. M. Caswell, M. Singh, and M. A. Persinger, "Simulated Sudden Increase in Geomagnetic Activity and Its Effect on Heart Rate Variability: Experimental Verification of Correlation Studies," *Life Sciences in Space Research* (2016), doi: 10.1016/j.lssr.2016.08.001; H. Mavromichalaki, P. Preka-Papadema, A. Theodoropoulou, et al., "A Study of the Possible Relation of the Cardiac Arrhythmias Occurrence to the Polarity Reversal of the Solar Magnetic Field," *Advances in Space Research* (2017), doi: 10.1016/j.asr.2016.08.024; R. McCraty, M. Atkinson, V. Stolc, et al., "Synchronization of Human Autonomic Nervous System Rhythms with Geomagnetic Activity in Human Subjects," *International Journal of Environmental Research and Public Health* (2017), doi: 10.3390/ijerph14070770; S. Ghione, L. Mezzasalma, C. Del Seppia, et al., "Do Geomagnetic Disturbances of Solar Origin Affect Arterial Blood Pressure?" *Journal of Human Hypertension* (1998), doi: 10.1038/sj.jhh.1000708; G. Chevalier, S. Patel, L. Weiss, et al., "The Effects of Grounding (Earthing) on Bodyworkers' Pain and Overall Quality of Life: A Randomized Controlled Trial," *Explore* (2019), doi: 10.1016/j.explore.2018.10.001; G. Chevalier, S. T. Sinatra, J. L. Oschman, et al., "Earthing: Health Implications of Reconnecting the Human Body to the Earth's Surface Electrons," *Journal of*

Environmental and Public Health (2012), doi: 10.1155/2012/291541; G. Chevalier, K. Mori, and J. L. Oschman, "The Effect of Earthing (Grounding) on Human Physiology," *European Biology and Bioelectromagnetics* (2006); J. L. Oschman, G. Chevalier, and R. Brown, "The Effects of Grounding (Earthing) on Inflammation, the Immune Response, Wound Healing, and Prevention and Treatment of Chronic Inflammatory and Autoimmune Diseases," *Journal of Inflammation Research* (2015), doi: 10.2147/JIR.S69656.

4. G. Chevalier, R. Brown, and M. Hill, "Grounding after Moderate Eccentric Contractions Reduces Muscle Damage," *Open Access Journal of Sports Medicine* (2015), doi: 10.2147/oajsm.s87970.

5. R. Passi, K. K. Doheny, Y. Gordin, et al., "Electrical Grounding Improves Vagal Tone in Preterm Infants," *Neonatology* (2017), doi: 10.1159/000475744.

Chapter 11: Flow with Emotional Energy

1. M. Kozela, M. Bobak, A. Besala, et al., "The Association of Depressive Symptoms with Cardiovascular and All-Cause Mortality in Central and Eastern Europe: Prospective Results of the HAPIEE Study," *European Journal of Preventive Cardiology* (2016), doi: 10.1177/2047487316649493; H. Fan, W. Yu, Q. Zhang, et al., "Depression after Heart Failure and Risk of Cardiovascular and All-Cause Mortality: A Meta-Analysis," *Preventive Medicine* (2014), doi: 10.1016 /j.ypmed.2014.03.007; M. Majd and E. E. C. Saunders, "Inflammation and the Dimensions of Depression: A Review," *Frontiers in Neuroendocrinology* (2019), doi: 10.1016/j.yfrne.2019.100800.

2. T. W. Smith, B. N. Uchino, J. A. Bosch, et al., "Trait Hostility Is Associated with Systemic Inflammation in Married Couples: An Actor-Partner Analysis," *Biological Psychology* (2014), doi: 10.1016/j.biopsycho.2014.07.005; S. Jain, J. E. Dimsdale, S. C. Roesch, et al., "Ethnicity, Social Class, and Hostility: Effects on In Vivo Beta-Adrenergic Receptor Responsiveness," *Biological Psychology* 65, no. 2 (2004): 89–100, doi: 10.1016/S0301-0511(03)00111-X; J. E. Graham, T. F. Robles, J. K. Kiecolt-Glaser, et al., "Hostility and Pain Are Related to Inflammation in Older Adults," *Brain, Behavior, and Immunity* (2006), doi: 10.1016/j.bbi.2005.11.002; D. Janicki-Deverts, S. Cohen, and W. J. Doyle, "Cynical Hostility and Stimulated Th1 and Th2 Cytokine Production," *Brain, Behavior, and Immunity* (2010), doi: 10.1016/j.bbi.2009.07.009; D. Kim, L. D. Kubzansky, A. Baccarelli, et al., "Psychological Factors and DNA Methylation of Genes Related to Immune/ Inflammatory System Markers: The VA Normative Aging Study," *BMJ Open* 6, no. 1 (2016): e009790, doi: 10.1136/bmjopen-2015-009790; J. Boisclair Demarble, D. S. Moskowitz, J. C. Tardif, et al., "The Relation Between Hostility and Concurrent Levels of Inflammation Is Sex, Age, and Measure Dependent," *Journal of Psychosomatic Research* (2014), doi: 10.1016/j.jpsychores.2014.02.010.

3. C. Albus, "Psychological and Social Factors in Coronary Heart Disease," *Annals of Medicine* (2010), doi: 10.3109/07853890.2010.515605; T. Q. Miller, T. W. Smith,

C. W. Turner, et al., "A Meta-Analytic Review of Research on Hostility and Physical Health," *Psychological Bulletin* (1996), doi: 10.1037/0033-2909.119.2.322.

4. J. T. Moskowitz, E. S. Epel, and M. Acree, "Positive Affect Uniquely Predicts Lower Risk of Mortality in People with Diabetes," *Health Psychology* 27, no. 1, Suppl. (2008): S73–S82, doi: 10.1037/0278-6133.27.1.S73; J. T. Moskowitz, "Positive Affect Predicts Lower Risk of AIDS Mortality," *Psychosomatic Medicine* 65, no. 4 (2003): 620–626, doi: 10.1097/01.PSY.0000073873.74829.23; Y. Chida and A. Steptoe, "Positive Psychological Well-Being and Mortality: A Quantitative Review of Prospective Observational Studies," *Psychosomatic Medicine* 70, no. 7 (2008): 741–756, doi: 10.1097/PSY.0b013e31818105ba.

5. S. D. Pressman and L. L. Black, "Positive Emotions and Immunity," in *The Oxford Handbook of Psychoneuroimmunology* (Oxford, UK: Oxford University Press, 2012), doi: 10.1093/oxfordhb/9780195394399.013.0006.

6. P. Cuijpers, A. van Straten, and L. Warmerdam, "Behavioral Activation Treatments of Depression: A Meta-Analysis," *Clinical Psychology Review* 27, no. 3 (2007): 318–326, doi: 10.1016/j.cpr.2006.11.001.

7. J. H. Fowler and N. A. Christakis, "Dynamic Spread of Happiness in a Large Social Network: Longitudinal Analysis over 20 Years in the Framingham Heart Study," *BMJ* 338, no. 7685 (2009): 1–13, doi: 10.1136/bmj.a2338.

8. A. D. I. Kramer, J. E. Guillory, and J. T. Hancock, "Experimental Evidence of Massive-Scale Emotional Contagion Through Social Networks," *Proceedings of the National Academy of Sciences of the United States of America* 111, no. 24 (2014): 8788–8790, doi: 10.1073/pnas.1320040111.

9. F. Borgonovi, "Doing Well by Doing Good: The Relationship Between Formal Volunteering and Self-Reported Health and Happiness," *Social Science and Medicine* 66, no. 11 (2008): 2321–2334, doi: 10.1016/j.socscimed.2008.01.011.

Chapter 12: Express Your Creativity to Jump-Start Vitality

1. H. L. Stuckey and J. Nobel, "The Connection Between Art, Healing, and Public Health: A Review of Current Literature," *American Journal of Public Health* (2010), doi: 10.2105/AJPH.2008.156497.

2. J. Berman, "The Writing Cure: How Expressive Writing Promotes Health and Emotional Well-Being," *Psychoanalytic Psychology* (2003), doi: 10.1037/0736-9735.20.3.575.

3. S. B. Kaufman, "The Neuroscience of Creativity: A Q and A with Anna Abraham," *Scientific American* (2019), blogs.scientificamerican.com/beautiful-minds/the-neuroscience-of-creativity-a-q-a-with-anna-abraham/.

4. A. A. Kaptein, B. M. Hughes, M. Murray, et al., "Start Making Sense: Art Informing Health Psychology," *Health Psychology Open* (2018), doi: 10.1177/2055102918760042.

5. M. Flood and K. D. Phillips, "Creativity in Older Adults: A Plethora of Possibilities," *Issues in Mental Health Nursing* (2007), doi: 10.1080/01612840701252956.

6. C. D. Ryff, B. H. Singer, and G. D. Love, "Positive Health: Connecting Well-Being with Biology," *Philosophical Transactions of the Royal Society B: Biological Sciences* (2004), doi: 10.1098/rstb.2004.1521.

7. T. S. Conner, C. G. DeYoung, and P. J. Silvia, "Everyday Creative Activity as a Path to Flourishing," *Journal of Positive Psychology* (2018), doi: 10.1080/17439760.2016.1257049.

8. C. Byrge and C. Tang, "Embodied Creativity Training: Effects on Creative Self-Efficacy and Creative Production," *Thinking Skills and Creativity* (2015), doi: 10.1016/j.tsc.2015.01.002; G. E. Mathisen and K. S. Bronnick, "Creative Self-Efficacy: An Intervention Study," *International Journal of Educational Research* (2009), doi: 10.1016/j.ijer.2009.02.009.

9. P. Siegel and N. F. Barros, "Religious Therapeutics, Body, and Health in Yoga, Ayurveda, and Tantra," *Ciência & Saúde Coletiva* (2007), doi: 10.1590/S1413 -81232007000600035; G. Feuerstein, *Tantra: The Path of Ecstacy* (Boston: Shambala, 1998); M. P. C. Toro, M. Á. Macías, and M. E. M. Pedroza, "Sexuality: From Taoism to Chinese Medicine" (2018), doi: 10.1016/j.acu.2018.07.001.

10. J. R. Averill, "Emotional Creativity: Toward 'Spiritualizing the Passions,'" in *The Oxford Handbook of Positive Psychology*, 2nd ed. (Oxford, UK: Oxford University Press, 2012), doi: 10.1093/oxfordhb/9780195187243.013.0023.

Chapter 13: Set Your Healing Intention Through Ritual

1. Z. Di Blasi, E. Harkness, E. Ernst, et al., "Influence of Context Effects on Health Outcomes: A Systematic Review," *Lancet* (2001), doi: 10.1016/S0140-6736(00) 04169-6.

2. M. V. Mondloch, D. C. Cole, and J. W. Frank, "Does How You Do Depend on How You Think You'll Do? A Systematic Review of the Evidence for a Relation Between Patients' Recovery Expectations and Health Outcomes," *Canadian Medical Association Journal* (2001).

3. B. Rutherford, T. Wager, and S. Roose, "Expectancy and the Treatment of Depression: A Review of Experimental Methodology and Effects on Patient Outcome," *Current Psychiatry Reviews* (2010), doi: 10.2174/157340010790596571; D. G. Finniss, T. J. Kaptchuk, F. Miller, et al., "Placebo Effects: Biological, Clinical, and Ethical Advances," *Lancet* 375, no. 9715 (2010): 686–695, doi: 10.1016/S0140 -6736(09)61706-2; R. Klinger, J. Stuhlreyer, M. Schwartz, et al., "Clinical Use of Placebo Effects in Patients with Pain Disorders," *International Review of Neurobiology* (2018), doi: 10.1016/bs.irn.2018.07.015.

4. Finniss, Kaptchuk, Miller, et al., "Placebo Effects."

5. M. Amanzio and F. Benedetti, "Neuropharmacological Dissection of Placebo Analgesia: Expectation-Activated Opioid Systems Versus Conditioning-Activated Specific Subsystems," *Journal of Neuroscience* 19, no. 1 (1999): 484–494, doi: 10.1038/nrn3465; F. Benedetti, "Mechanisms of Placebo and Placebo-Related Effects Across Diseases and Treatments," *Annual Review of Pharmacology and Toxicology* (2008), doi: 10.1146/annurev.pharmtox.48.113006.094711.

6. D. D. Price, D. G. Finniss, and F. Benedetti, "A Comprehensive Review of the Placebo Effect: Recent Advances and Current Thought," *Annual Review of Psychology* (2008), doi: 10.1146/annurev.psych.59.113006.095941; F. Benedetti, E. Carlino, and A. Pollo, "How Placebos Change the Patient's Brain," *Neuropsychopharmacology* 36, no. 1 (2011): 339–354, doi: 10.1038/npp.2010.81; R. De la Fuente-Fernández, A. G. Phillips, M. Zamburlini, et al., "Dopamine Release in Human Ventral Striatum and Expectation of Reward," *Behavioural Brain Research* (2002), doi: 10.1016/S0166-4328(02)00130-4; R. De la Fuente-Fernández, T. J. Ruth, V. Sossi, et al., "Expectation and Dopamine Release: Mechanism of the Placebo Effect in Parkinson's Disease," *Science* (2001), doi: 10.1126/science.1060937; A. Strafella, "Therapeutic Application of Transcranial Magnetic Stimulation in Parkinson's Disease: The Contribution of Expectation," *NeuroImage* (2006), doi: 10.1016/j.neuroimage.2006.02.005.

7. J. Daubenmier, D. Chopra, S. Jain, et al., "Indo-Tibetan Philosophical and Medical Systems: Perspectives on the Biofield," *Global Advances in Health and Medicine* (2015), doi: 10.7453/gahmj.2015.026.suppl.; R. Gombrich, review of "Middle Indo-Aryan and Jaina Studies," ed. C. Caillat, in *Sanskrit Outside India*, ed. J. G. de Casparis, Panels of the VIIth World Sanskrit Conference, Kern Institute, Leiden, August 23–29, 1987, vols. 6–7 (Leiden: E. J. Brill, 1991), in *Journal of the Royal Asiatic Society* 3, no. 2 (1993): 288–290, doi: 10.1017/S1356186300004569.

8. S. S. Sivananda, *The Science of Pranayama* (Bartolini, Italy: Youcanprint.it, 2017).

9. S. S. Goswami, *Layayoga: The Definitive Guide to the Chakras and Kundalini* (Rochester, VT: Inner Traditions, 1999).

10. D. Frawley, *Mantra Yoga and the Primal Sound: Secrets of Seed (Bija) Mantras* (Detroit: Lotus, 2010).

11. John 1, *New King James Version*, Bible Gateway.

12. M. Winkleman, "Shamanism and the Origins of Spirituality and Ritual Healing," *Journal for the Study of Religion, Nature, and Culture* 3, no. 4 (2010): 458–489, doi: 10.1558/jsrnc.v3i4.458.

13. M. A. Winkelman, "Cross-Cultural Study of Shamanistic Healers," *Journal of Psychoactive Drugs* 21, no. 1 (1989): 17–24, doi: 10.1080/02791072.1989.10472139.

14. J. Levin, "Energy Healers: Who They Are and What They Do," *Explore* 7, no. 1 (2011): 13–26, doi: 10.1016/j.explore.2010.10.005.

Chapter 14: Connect to Heal

1. H. V. Fineberg, "Pandemic Preparedness and Response: Lessons from the H1N1 Influenza of 2009," *New England Journal of Medicine* 370, no. 14 (2014): 1335–1342, doi: 10.1056/NEJMra1208802.

2. J. T. Cacioppo and W. Patrick, *Loneliness: Human Nature and the Need for Social Connection* (New York: Norton, 2008).

3. J. Holt-Lunstad, T. Robles, and D. A. Sbarra, "Advancing Social Connection as a Public Health Priority in the United States," *American Psychology* 72, no. 6 (2017):

517–530, doi: 10.1037/amp0000103; D. Umberson and J. Karas Montez, "Social Relationships and Health: A Flashpoint for Health Policy," *Journal of Health and Social Behavavior* 51, Suppl. (2010): S54–S66, doi: 10.1177/0022146510383501.

4. J. Holt-Lunstad, T. B. Smith, and J. B. Layton, "Social Relationships and Mortality Risk: A Meta-Analytic Review," *PLoS Medicine* 7, no. 7 (2010), doi: 10.1371/journal.pmed.1000316.

5. B. N. Uchino, "Social Support and Health: A Review of Physiological Processes Potentially Underlying Links to Disease Outcomes," *Journal of Behavioral Medicine* 29, no. 4 (2006): 377–387, doi: 10.1007/s10865-006-9056-5.

6. S. Kennedy, J. K. Kiecolt-Glaser, and R. Glaser, "Social Support, Stress, and the Immune System," in *Social Support: An Interactional View* (Hoboken, NJ: Wiley, 1990), 253–266.

7. C. L. Carmichael, H. T. Reis, and P. R. Duberstein, "In Your 20s It's Quantity; in Your 30s It's Quality: The Prognostic Value of Social Activity Across 30 Years of Adulthood," *Psychology and Aging* 30, no. 1 (2015): 95–105, doi: 10.1037/pag0000014.

8. N. I. Eisenberger, M. D. Lieberman, and K. D. Williams, "Does Rejection Hurt? An FMRI Study of Social Exclusion," *Science* 302, no. 5643 (2003): 290–292, doi: 10.1126/science.1089134; N. I. Eisenberger, "The Pain of Social Disconnection: Examining the Shared Neural Underpinnings of Physical and Social Pain," *Nature Reviews Neuroscience* 13, no. 6 (2012): 421–434, doi: 10.1038/nrn3231.

9. K. J. Kemper and H. A. Shaltout, "Non-Verbal Communication of Compassion: Measuring Psychophysiologic Effects," *BMC Complementary and Alternative Medicine* 11 (2011): 132, doi: 10.1186/1472-6882-11-132.

10. A. Sieber, "Hanh's Concept of Being Peace: The Order of Interbeing," *International Journal of Religion and Spirituality in Society* 5, no. 1 (2015): 1–8, doi: 10.18848/2154-8633/CGP/v05i01/51097.

11. J. Pérez-Remón, *Self and Non-Self in Early Buddhism* (Berlin: de Gruyter, 2012).

12. Y. Dor-Ziderman, A. Berkovich-Ohana, J. Glicksohn, et al., "Mindfulness-Induced Selflessness: A MEG Neurophenomenological Study," *Frontiers in Human Neuroscience* 7 (2013): 582, doi: 10.3389/fnhum.2013.00582; N. E. Rosenthal, *Transcendence: Healing and Transformation Through Transcendental Meditation* (New York: Penguin, 2012); S. Young, "Purpose and Method of Vipassana Meditation," *Humanistic Psychologist* 22, no. 1 (1994): 53–61, doi: 10.1080/08873267.1994.9976936.

13. P. Oehen, R. Traber, V. Widmer, et al., "A Randomized, Controlled Pilot Study of MDMA (±3,4-Methylenedioxymethamphetamine)-Assisted Psychotherapy for Treatment of Resistant, Chronic Post-Traumatic Stress Disorder (PTSD)," *Journal of Psychopharmacology* 27, no. 1 (2013): 43–52, doi: 10.1177/0269881112464827.

Chapter 15: Surrender

1. J. Nowinski, "Facilitating 12-Step Recovery from Substance Abuse and Addiction," in *Treating Substance Abuse: Theory and Technique*, 2nd ed. (New York: Guilford, 2003), 31–66; D. Berenson, "Alcoholics Anonymous: From Surrender to Transformation," *Family Therapy Networker* 11, no. 4 (1987): 24–31; R. P. Speer, "Surrender and Recovery," *Alcoholism Treatment Quarterly* 16, no. 4 (1999): 21–29, doi: 10.1300/J020v16n04_03; H. M. Tiebout, *The Ego Factors in Surrender in Alcoholism* (New York: National Council on Alcoholism, 1954); D. G. Benner, *Surrender to Love: Discovering the Heart of Christian Spirituality* (Westmont, IL: InterVarsity Press, 2015); F. X. Clooney, *Beyond Compare: St. Francis de Sales and Sri Vedanta Desika on Loving Surrender to God* (Washington, DC: Georgetown University Press; 2008).

2. A. D. Clements and A. V. Ermakova, "Surrender to God and Stress: A Possible Link Between Religiosity and Health," *Psychology of Religion and Spirituality* 4, no. 2 (2012): 93–107, doi: 10.1037/a0025109; A. Wong-Mcdonald and R. L. Gorsuch, "Surrender to God: An Additional Coping Style?" *Journal of Psychology and Theology* 28, no. 2 (2000): 149–161, doi: 10.1177/009164710002800207; L. Rosequist, K. Wall, D. Corwin, et al., "Surrender as a Form of Active Acceptance Among Breast Cancer Survivors Receiving Psycho-Spiritual Integrative Therapy," *Supportive Care in Cancer* 20, no. 11 (2012): 2821–2827, doi: 10.1007/s00520-012-1406-y.

3. T. Frederick and K. M. White, "Mindfulness, Christian Devotion Meditation, Surrender, and Worry," *Mental Health, Religion, and Culture* 18, no. 10 (2015): 850–858, doi: 10.1080/13674676.2015.1107892.

4. S. S. Goswami, *Layayoga: The Definitive Guide to the Chakras and Kundalini* (Rochester, VT: Inner Traditions, 1999); K. Leland, *Rainbow Body: A History of the Western Chakra System from Blavatsky to Brennan* (Newburyport, MA: Red Wheel/Weiser, 2016).

5. R. Fischer, "A Cartography of the Ecstatic and Meditative States," *Science* 174, no. 4012 (1971): 29.

INDEX

ABOUT THE AUTHOR

Shamini Jain, PhD, is a psychologist, scientist, and social entrepreneur. She is the founder and CEO of the Consciousness and Healing Initiative (CHI), a nonprofit, collaborative accelerator that connects scientists, health practitioners, educators, and artists to help lead humanity to heal ourselves. CHI was formed through Dr. Jain's deep desire to bring key stakeholders together to create a coherent and effective movement in order to move us beyond models of disease thinking and medical management into the study of systems-based healing and personal and societal empowerment. Dr. Jain also serves as adjunct faculty at UC San Diego, where she is an active member of the UC San Diego Center for Integrative Medicine's research committee.

Dr. Jain obtained her BA degree in Neuroscience and Behavior at Columbia University, her MA degree in Integrative Health Psychology from the University of Arizona, and her PhD in Clinical Psychology and Psychoneuroimmunology from the San Diego State University/UC San Diego joint doctoral program in Clinical Psychology. She conducted her clinical internship at the Veterans Affairs (VA) Medical Center in La Jolla, CA, and her post-doctoral fellowship at UCLA's Center of Cancer Prevention and Control Research. Dr. Jain has received numerous awards for her pioneering research in meditation, biofield healing, and psychoneuroimmunology, which has been featured in *TIME, US News and World Report,* CNN, and other news media.

Dr. Jain is an international keynote speaker and teacher. She integrates her background in clinical psychology, psychoneuroimmunology, Jainst spiritual wisdom, and the healing arts in order to teach people how they can best heal themselves and live life with joy and spiritual alignment on purpose. She teaches regularly in retreat centers, including Esalen and Kripalu, and shares her research on the science of healing in diverse venues, including NATO, TEDx, major universities and medical centers, health-related conferences, and corporations.

Dr. Jain is a member of the Evolutionary Leaders Circle and serves as a board member and advisor for several nonprofit and social benefit companies, including Greenheart, Modern Spirit, Wacuri, and Leap Forward. Beyond forwarding the science and practice of healing, her biggest joys are spending time with her beautiful family, singing, and surfing. Learn more at chi.is and shaminijain.com.

ABOUT SOUNDS TRUE

Sounds True is a multimedia publisher whose mission is to inspire and support personal transformation and spiritual awakening. Founded in 1985 and located in Boulder, Colorado, we work with many of the leading spiritual teachers, thinkers, healers, and visionary artists of our time. We strive with every title to preserve the essential "living wisdom" of the author or artist. It is our goal to create products that not only provide information to a reader or listener but also embody the quality of a wisdom transmission.

For those seeking genuine transformation, Sounds True is your trusted partner. At SoundsTrue.com you will find a wealth of free resources to support your journey, including exclusive weekly audio interviews, free downloads, interactive learning tools, and other special savings on all our titles.

To learn more, please visit SoundsTrue.com/freegifts or call us toll-free at 800.333.9185.

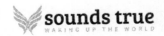

sounds true
WAKING UP THE WORLD